Happy Naturally

A QUICK GUIDE TO
SUPPLEMENTS AND SELF-HELP TOOLS
FOR DEPRESSION AND ANXIETY

Happy
Naturally

Raphael Allred, M.D.

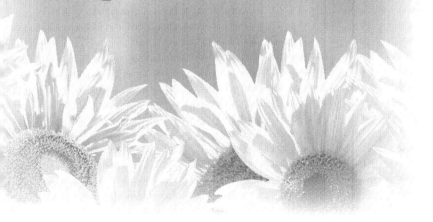

Note: The information in this book is factual and true to the best of the author's knowledge and is not intended to replace regular medical care or contradict advice from your physician. Please use common sense as well as guidance from your physician when making choices regarding your health. The information in this book is offered in general and without guarantees. In the event that you use any of the information in this book for yourself, the author and publisher assume no liability for your actions. The author was not paid by any company to promote products, services or resources.

A special THANK YOU to my parents, my patients and my children for all you have taught me.

This book is dedicated to my husband.
Thank you for being my rock, for loving me and
for showing me how to become the best possible me.

Table of Contents

PART 2 MENTAL

PART 3 EMOTIONAL

PART 4 THE SPECIAL CIRCUMSTANCES

SUPPLEMENTS

ADDITIONAL RESOURCES

BIBLIOGRAPHY

Introduction

Do you ever wonder why you struggle to feel happy? Why you lost that joy for life that you had when you were younger? Or are you someone who doesn't remember a time when you felt happy? You aren't alone. So many of us struggle with depression at one point or another, and unfortunately many people suffer alone because they are too embarrassed to seek help, viewing their depression as a weakness that they should overcome on their own.

It may be that you are someone who has asked for help, has taken medications in the past, or is currently on a medication but is looking for other options. Medications have their time and place but they also have the potential for unwanted side effects as well as embarrassment that some feel about taking an antidepressant.

I've always had a keen interest in depression and anxiety, having dealt with them personally since I was a child. I remember having stomach aches daily before school and feeling tightness in my chest walking to the bus stop. When I got older I fantasized about driving away without telling anyone where I was going, and moving to a small town in the middle of nowhere. Logically I knew that big cities are better places to hide, but they give me anxiety...so small town it was. Clearly I couldn't escape that easily so I learned coping strategies, but it's been a lifelong quest to find better and more effective tools to bring peace and happiness into my life. In the last fifteen years of practice as a family physician this has become a major area of interest for me as I've seen so many patients struggle with depression and anxiety.

Depression and anxiety are complex topics and volumes have been written about each. I am choosing to keep it simple. This book isn't meant to be a comprehensive scientific or medical guide to all treatments for depression and anxiety. Rather, it is a way for me to share what I've learned on my personal journey with anxiety and depression, both as a woman and as a physician. I won't be quoting the latest studies or medical articles, since you can easily look those up online, but rather will be sharing what has worked for me and my patients. You may have chosen this book because you are on a journey to wellness—not just physical, but emotional and mental health as well. There is no one thing in this life that will give you instant wellness. It's a journey, not a destination, and will take you down many paths of healing, and I'm so happy to be part of your quest for happiness and health.

Throughout this book I may refer to depression and anxiety interchangeably. They are not the same but often go hand in hand when serotonin levels are low. I will talk more about serotonin later, but basically it's your "happy chemical" that regulates your mood. If it's too low then you can feel either depressed or anxious. If I talk about depression and you are only dealing with anxiety, just realize that the information often will apply to both situations. There is a section toward the end of the book you can reference that is devoted exclusively to anxiety.

Health is not only the absence of disease just as happiness is not merely the absence of depression. To be truly happy and healthy, we must be well, in mind, body and spirit. Depression is not just a physical change that happens in the brain, it is also the mental habits that affect our thoughts and mindset as well as our emotional state that tugs us into a downward spiral. Treating only one of these three key areas will leave us struggling to be happy and healthy. I have watched patients over the years leave with only a prescription in hand, declining any help with the mental or emotional aspect of their depression, only to return later frustrated with their lack of happiness. Addressing the emotional and mental component of depression, although difficult, is as important as the medications used to treat the physical changes happening in the brain.

The emphasis of this book is on non-pharmacological treatments, meaning everything except prescription strength medications. I believe that this country is over-medicated—that we doctors are too quick to put patients on anti-depressants or tranquilizers and leave them on medications for far too long. That being said, there are circumstance that call for pharmaceuticals and I am grateful to have them as a resource for my patients who have severe anxiety, suicidal thoughts or haven't improved with alternative treatment options. If you are currently taking a prescription antidepressant, please do NOT stop taking it cold turkey or without consulting your physician. This book is not intended to replace the care you receive from your physician. Instead, it is meant to be a complementary tool to give you hope, guidance and insight.

If you are reading this, then most likely your life has been touched by anxiety or depression, either your own or that of a loved one. I have a special place in my heart for you, knowing the lonely road you've been on so far. Please know you aren't alone and that you don't have to stay where you are. Turn the page and explore possibilities.

PART 1
PHYSICAL

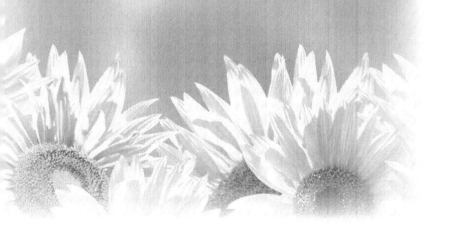

Chapter 1
The Basics of Depression and Anxiety

You may be a fortunate person who has never suffered from depression or anxiety, but it's likely you know someone who has. I recently looked at the statistics reported by both the CDC and the Anxiety and Depression Association of America. Between 5 percent and 18 percent of people suffer from either depression or anxiety right now. That doesn't take into account people who have suffered in the past and have pulled themselves through into a more happy and peaceful state. When I was in residency one of my fabulous mentors told me that 50 percent of family practice patients who seek care for any reason are suffering from some sort of mental or emotional illness. I've found that to be absolutely true—much more of disease is rooted in our mental state than we realize. It's impossible to be truly well physically without also having emotional and mental wellness. Depression and anxiety are two of the most common diagnoses I see in Family Medicine, and they affect every aspect of our lives: physical health, relationships, work

WHAT IS DEPRESSION?

Officially depression is a mood disorder that looks like prolonged sadness coupled with a loss of interest that affects normal daily function. It's often accompanied by changes in appetite, sleep, energy, libido and pain levels. Okay, that was the very technical definition. What does all that mean? It means you feel like you've fallen into a deep, dark hole that you will be alone in for the rest of your life. It feels like a crushing sadness for no clear reason. You feel guilty all the time. Your confidence is low because you feel like a loser and your thoughts are consistently negative, especially about yourself. You avoid people and events because they either exhaust you or you feel inadequate. Depression is not fun. At all.

Some people wonder, "Am I depressed?" This may sound silly, because isn't it obvious when you are depressed? No, not necessarily. It's normal to feel sad at times, even for prolonged periods such as during grief, but that doesn't necessarily constitute clinical depression. Depression can sneak up on you, since you can become used to feeling down and overwhelmed, and only by taking a step back and really evaluating can you see the situation clearly. My first year of medical practice I didn't realize why I was struggling to get out of bed in the mornings and wanted to sleep all the time. One day I gave my patient a depression screening tool and casually answered the questions for myself as I was waiting for her to finish. My score explained a lot about what was going on with me and was a bit of a wake-up call for me. I realized I was technically depressed and needed to do something about it. Had I not asked myself those questions I would have continued to just live with my symptoms. There are simple screening tools online, and the two most effective questions to start with are "have you found that you have little or no interest in doing the things you normally love?" and "have you been feeling down, hopeless or depressed?" You can get online and look at some other screening tools such as the Hamilton Depression Scale that will screen for symptoms of depression that aren't always obvious, but it is important to talk to your doctor about depression screening if you are feeling sad, down or hopeless.

Some of you reading this are thinking, "Well, I'm not depressed but I wish my spouse/partner/child/parent would realize they need some help." Unfortunately walking up to someone and saying, "I think you're depressed," doesn't usually yield the results we are hoping for. They have to want help, and you can gently point out the issue by asking them how they are feeling or by saying, "Hey, I was just reading about this interesting screening tool that is just two questions."

Depression affects not only our mental and emotional health, but also our physical health. That is not a surprise since they are intrinsically linked. For years I struggled with extreme fatigue as well as gut issues, joint pain, and headaches. These issues were intimately tied to how depressed or anxious I was feeling. People with chronic illnesses do worse when they are depressed, just as depressed people often develop physical illnesses. I have seen so many patients over the years with auto-immune diseases who have flares when they become depressed. Patients who have had a heart attack or stroke are significantly more likely to become depressed than the average person.

You will feel so much better physically when you feel your best emotionally and mentally. The same can be said of your relationships. They will thrive if you are doing well emotionally and they will suffer if you are struggling. My husband has been a source of strength and inspiration over the years and he has had to exercise great patience at times when I've been my most down. During one of my most depressed times he was trying to help cheer me up but I wasn't feeling validated. I reminded him that he has no idea how hard it is to feel depressed, but he reminded me that I have no idea how hard it is being married to a depressed person. It was exhausting for both of us.

It's also hard to be productive at work or at home when you are depressed, especially because you feel physically and mentally drained. I had a friend describe it this way: "I sit here on my couch and I see the clothes that need to be folded and the dishes that need to be washed, but the thought of getting up and doing them is overwhelming." I have had patients fall behind on their bills because the thought of opening mail or writing checks was too daunting. I've seen people lose their jobs because they just couldn't pull it together at work to complete tasks and deliver good customer service.

I'm sharing these things, not to be a downer but rather to help you realize that depression is not just a mental attitude or a physical condition. It a mixture of both and it affects much of our lives. The good news is that we don't have to stay there, that there are options, and you can be happy. Naturally.

WHAT IS ANXIETY?

There are several different types of anxiety, including post-traumatic s tress disorder, phobias, generalized anxiety disorder and anxiety that is a symptom of depression. I will talk more about anxiety later, but for now I'm going to keep it simple and talk about the anxiety seen commonly with depression. Think of serotonin "deficiency" as a two-sided coin with depression on one side and anxiety on the other. Anxiety usually involves the emotional feelings of anxiety and dread as well as the physical symptoms that come from that dread and anxiety. You know the feeling you get if you drink too much caffeine or if you have a crazy amount of stress in your life? That is what anxious people feel all the time, but often they don't know why. It's not logical and is very much related to the same brain chemistry changes that cause depression. Having both the sadness of depression and the dread of anxiety together is exhausting and disheartening.

Everyone feels stressed at times, everyone worries and many people are a bit high strung. True anxiety is all of those things but it's chronic and constant and makes daily functioning difficult, just as depression does. The difference is usually that depressed people tend to withdraw and feel down, whereas anxious people may unintentionally spill their tense energy onto the people around them. Again, I will talk more about anxiety later but if you are struggling with feeling nervous, anxious, stressed, or have a daily feeling of dread then you are likely dealing with anxiety. The good news is that awareness comes before change and we will talk about tools available to you.

The last thing I will say is that there are many people who don't want to address their depression or anxiety because of the stigma that is still attached to mental illness. If you thought you had high blood pressure or diabetes you would get the care you need. Unfortunately people often ignore their mental and emotional states because they feel embarrassed to talk about it. My response to my patients is "Denial is as good as placebo." Of course that is my joking response, but really, you can only progress in life when you acknowledge there is an issue in the first place. So kudos to you for realizing your starting point so we can move on from there.

HOW DID I END UP HERE?

I remember turning forty, looking at my life and feeling guilty for feeling depressed. I had a new baby, two other gorgeous kids, a wonderful husband, a successful medical practice and a supportive community. Why would I feel depressed? For me it was a combination of things. I was physically exhausted from poor sleep and hard work, the conflict of being a working mom and realizing that my life had settled into a rut. I was out of the exciting childbearing years, I had no new plans on the horizon for work, and I had "arrived" to my life as it would be for the foreseeable future. My world at that point didn't resemble the exciting life I had planned when I was younger, and worse, I had gotten complacent and comfortable. I was missing my fire and passion.

I think this is common, which is why so many people have midlife crises. We often feel that where we are is far from where we want to be. Dr. Seuss described it as the "waiting place" in his classic Oh The Places You'll Go. It is disconcerting to realize that is where you have landed, and it can lead to impulsive actions as well as depression. We'll talk more later about getting out of this place.

This isn't the only thing, of course, that can lead to depression. I want to pause here for a moment and talk about the chemical changes in a depressed brain. It will be short and painless and I will even throw in a couple of my diagrams to make it more interesting. First I will say that I'm going to dramatically oversimplify this explanation, but that's what makes it fun. Second, I will say that I'm going to focus on serotonin, that chemical messenger or neurotransmitter I mentioned earlier, but be aware that there are many other chemicals in our brain that play a part such as dopamine, norepinephrine and so on. I'm not going to get too detailed, though. I want to focus on how serotonin levels are critical to a healthy mental state.

Imagine you have a kitchen sink in your brain. The faucet drips serotonin into the sink, where it sits, waiting to be used by your brain to help keep things steady—your mood, libido, energy, anxiety control, pain control, concentration, sleep and appetite, to name a few. The sink also has a garbage disposal that grinds up the serotonin and recycles some of the parts back up to the faucet to make more serotonin. Some of the key ingredients for making and regulating serotonin are Zinc, Inositol, Vitamin B6, Folate and a form of tryptophan called 5HTP. If you don't have enough of these key ingredients, your serotonin production goes down, or your faucet drips much more slowly than your garbage disposal is grinding. That will cause a drop in your serotonin levels. I will talk later about ways to increase the rate of your serotonin production or "turn the faucet

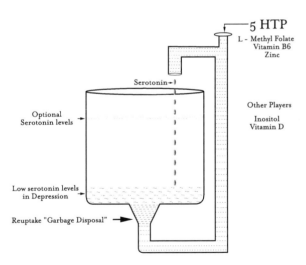

The Sink in our Brain

up higher" by getting more of the key ingredients to your brain. The other way to manipulate serotonin levels is by putting a stopper in your garbage disposal with a type of medication called an SSRI-selective serotonin reuptake inhibitor. No, there will not be a quiz later, but I just want you to be aware of how the most common antidepressants such as Prozac, Paxil, Zoloft and Lexapro work. When I refer to SSRI later in the book, I'm talking about this specific type of antidepressant that boosts your serotonin levels. But why do we have low serotonin levels at all?

LOW SEROTONIN

Some people have a genetic predisposition to a low level of serotonin. In those families you will often see a history of depression, suicide, alcoholism or another addiction. In my personal and professional experience, those of us with that genetic predisposition tend to become depressed very easily compared to the average population.

I also see depression very commonly during a major life change—both positive and negative changes. It's no surprise that losing a job, going bankrupt, getting a divorce, losing a loved one or becoming an empty nester can trigger depression, to name a few of the tough changes in life. But good changes can also cause major drops in our serotonin levels as the brain dips into our sink in an effort to keep things stable. Starting college, getting married, having a baby, moving or even starting a new career can trigger depression because they are such major changes. I remember being terribly depressed after I got married. Come to think of it, I've suffered depression with every major change in life—marriage, childbirth, starting my practice. I'm sure many of you can relate, and like me felt that bewildered guilt of wondering, "Why do I feel depressed when I should be feeling happy?"

HORMONES

Another factor is the effect of hormones on serotonin. There is a balance between serotonin, thyroid and the other hormones in our body and when one is too low or too high, the other two can be affected.

So what causes hormones to go haywire and mess up the balance of serotonin and other chemicals in our brain? Sometimes, like with premenstrual dysphoric disorder or PMS, it's a severe extreme of a normal cycle. It is normal for a woman to have a drop in her progesterone levels monthly, but with PMS the massive drops in progesterone levels the week before a menstrual period are so severe that there is a major mood change. Clearly menopause is another big trigger for hormone changes and it's not as simple as low estrogen and progesterone. The whole balance of hormones is disrupted.

We commonly think of estrogen and progesterone when we think of hormones, but testosterone and cortisol levels play a part as well.

Testosterone levels can fall with age or various medical conditions, which causes mood changes. Cortisol is our "stress hormone" that goes up in the morning to get us going and is supposed to go down in the evening to allow us to sleep. If it is too high then we feel snacky,

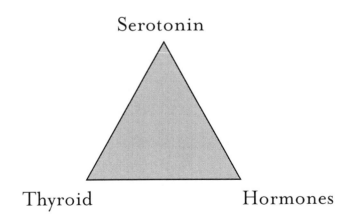

When one is off, the other two are impacted.

restless and sleep is hard to come by, which can affect serotonin levels. Chronic stress can wreak havoc with our hormone balance. Chronic stress causes higher levels of adrenaline and cortisol, both produced in the adrenal glands. When we are chronically stressed we can literally exhaust our adrenal glands, which then affects all the above hormones—which then affects the levels of serotonin in our brain.

Our thyroid is the last player in the hormone/serotonin/thyroid triangle. Think of your thyroid, the gland in your neck, as the thermostat for your body. It controls how slow or fast your metabolism is, which controls your weight and your temperature stability. If your thyroid is off then you may feel tired, constipated, gain weight and have mental fog, dry skin, and at times, depression. If you are like me, you would love the diagnosis of hypothyroidism so you could take one little pill a day and potentially lose weight and have more energy. It's definitely worth getting checked if you have some of the symptoms I just listed. Please ask your doctor to check all three thyroid levels, not just the thyroid stimulating hormone or TSH that is most commonly checked. I also feel it's important to directly check the levels of T3 and T4 as well. Replacing your thyroid hormone is simple and may change your life and greatly improve your depression.

MISSING INGREDIENTS

We've talked about the impact of genetics, life stressors and hormones on your mood, but there are other things that can lead to low serotonin. Remember the faucet in your brain that is dripping serotonin into your sink? Well, it has to have certain ingredients on hand in order to produce the serotonin. Think of baking a batch of cookies—you just can't do it if you are missing one of the ingredients. It's the same with our brain; if we don't have those essential vitamins, co-enzymes and minerals, then we don't get the levels of serotonin we need. Many times we just aren't eating enough of the right foods to get our necessary "ingredients." What are the right foods? You guessed it—fruits and vegetables are the biggest nutrient source we need. Not just any fruit or vegetable, either—the more colorful, the better. If it stains your clothing, it is loaded with antioxidants, many of which are needed for serotonin production.

Now, if you are someone who eats a ton of fruits and vegetables and still struggles, then it's possible you aren't absorbing the nutrition you need from your food. There are a couple of different ways you can deal with this possible scenario. The first option is to talk to either your family doctor or a naturopath about checking your blood levels. This can be pricey if you actually check all your different vitamin and neurotransmitter levels, and most insurance won't cover all these tests.

Another option you have is to assume that your levels are low and that your gut health isn't optimal. This will affect how you absorb your nutrition so you can try taking a high quality probiotic for two months and see how you feel. With the toxins in our foods, the low nutritional density of foods, and frequent antibiotic use, many of us have compromised gut absorption. That isn't even addressing medical conditions such as celiac sprue or leaky gut syndrome, which are a whole different ball game.

Usually, though, a good diet combined with a probiotic will go a long way toward balancing brain chemistry. Do an experiment: focus on eating more fruits and veggies and cut out the processed food and sugar for three days, and see how your mood is doing. Or do the opposite and eat heavy foods loaded with carbs and sugar and fat and see how you do. Some foods will lighten your mood and some will make you feel down, but unfortunately when we are down or stressed we tend to reach for those mood lowering foods because they give us pleasure for a few seconds, but overall they make us feel far worse. You can read more about this in *The Antianxiety Food Solution*, by Trudy Scott.

The last thing I will touch on is folate "deficiency" caused by the MTHFR gene mutation.[1] Now don't panic and skip this section because I threw in some fancy science terminology—I promise to explain.

---

1. You can read more about this at https://ghr.nlm.nih.gov/gene/MTHFR

Remember how our brain needs folate to make serotonin? Folate is a B vitamin we are all familiar with because the synthetic folic acid is added to foods to ensure that women get it in their diets to prevent birth defects. The folate itself isn't used to make serotonin unless it's converted to something called L-methyl folate or methylated folate. Again, don't get bogged down in the names. Think of it this way: in order to go trailer camping you have to hitch a camper onto your truck or car. In order to use folate to make serotonin, your body has to "hitch" a methyl group onto the folate. The hitch your brain uses is the enzyme MTHFR, which is the mercifully short acronym for methylenetetrahydrafolate reducase. So if you have a mutation of the MTHFR gene then your body can't convert folate to L-methyl folate which means that you can't make serotonin. Yes, this is an oversimplification, but it helps me explain what causes many people to feel depressed and anxious even if they are doing all the right things and taking all the right medications. The methylated folate is a key ingredient in your serotonin production, so it's clearly a problem if you have a MTHFR gene mutation. This can be inherited from one or both of your parents, but like any gene mutation, it's possible that stress or environmental pollutants play a role. The exact percentage of people with MTHFR gene mutation isn't well known because we are just now starting to test for it more regularly. Because the blood test for this condition isn't always covered by insurance and runs from $200–$400 depending upon the lab, I often have patients take a methylated folate supplement for a few weeks to see how they feel. If their mood improves then I think it's worth staying on the supplement. More on this supplement later.

As you can see, depression isn't caused by one isolated thing. It can be very complex, with both physical and emotional factors, and starting down the road to peace and happiness is sometimes daunting. In the next chapter I'm going to cover a few things you can do to address the physical aspect of the depression—things that will help raise your serotonin levels and get you farther down the path on your journey to wellness.

Chapter 2
Changing Your Brain Chemistry

Have you ever done a Google search for natural treatments for depression? You will be bombarded with possibilities, and just because it's on the internet doesn't mean that it's accurate or that the source is credible. I've been slowly gathering information about "alternative" treatments for the past twenty years. Let me pause and note how interesting it is that non-prescription options are considered alternative, despite having been around for much longer than prescription medication, which was introduced a short 125 years or so ago. But whatever your view, it is still a lovely option to explore complementary treatments as an alternative or adjunct to standard medical recommendations. Again, I'm not advocating that you stop all your prescription medications abruptly or even at all, but it's definitely worth adding some natural options to boost the effects of your meds, wean off your meds, or help you avoid medications to begin with. Be sure to consult with your physician no matter which category you fall into, but let's look at some great tools for you to begin with now.

NUTRITION

In my opinion, the first and best thing you can do is to eat a healthy diet. Hippocrates stated it best when he said, "Let food be thy medicine and medicine be thy food." As a society we have certainly strayed from this philosophy. I look at my diet compared to that of my great-grandparents and it's vastly different. My diet is many steps removed from the earth, whereas theirs was much closer to the original plant or animal source. A great read on this topic is *In Defense of Food*, by Michael Pollan.

We often expect high performance from our bodies, but just like our cars, if we put average fuel in them we will get average or less than average performance. I tell my patients all the time that nutrition is the foundation of our health. The types of food we eat not only determine our energy but also affect our moods. For instance, eating empty calories in candy will satisfy a craving for a moment, but then leave you feeling heavy, and if you pay close attention you may notice that you feel down or edgy afterward. On the other hand, eating healthy whole foods of protein with veggies and a healthy grain will leave you feeling light and happy, unless you over eat, of course. No one feels great after overeating. My point here is that food not only has nutritional value but contributes energetically to how we are feeling. I read an article recently that discussed the link between nutrition and mental illness. Teens with poor nutrition had 80 percent higher rates of depression compared to teens with high quality diets, according to the article.[2] That is an appalling statistic.

Clearly nutrition in general is a huge issue but I feel there is a tendency to brush it off as not important. There are several documentaries that will raise your awareness of nutrition and the foods we eat. I was particularly appalled and fascinated by the information in Forks Over Knives and Food, Inc.

Now, I would love to say that I eat only raw, organic whole foods and never have processed or refined foods pass my lips. But then I would be a liar. Yes I feel this is optimal, and if you can do it then you deserve a pat on the back and a gold star for excellence. Most of us are too lazy, too busy or too weak to eat a perfect diet. I still focus

---

2. Miller, Kelli. "The Food-Mood Link." WebMD Mar.-Apr. 2016: 43. Print.

on getting a diet rich in fruits and veggies, but do I get enough and how nutritionally replete is the food we buy now? This is where good supplementation comes in play.

SUPPLEMENTS

I used to roll my eyes when asked about supplements because for too long they weren't regulated by the FDA and you had no idea what was really in your capsule, tablet or powder. I felt that people were being exploited by companies just trying to capitalize on the wellness and supplement trend. But then I had my own experience with what a really high quality supplement can do.

I've dealt with anxiety and depression since I was a child, but they got severe around the time I took my first job at a family practice clinic. I also got married that same year, which was another major adjustment as I had some unrealistic expectations about "happily ever after." That was the first time I went on a prescription drug. I started an SSRI and felt only slightly better, and ended up adding a second drug that targeted norepinephrine and dopamine. The two medications helped me feel more stable but also a bit numb, and it wasn't until I added counseling to the regimen that I actually made progress and was able to get off my meds. Fast forward a few years and I was struggling with major postpartum depression. After each delivery I took generic Zoloft for a short time, but after my third baby I couldn't seem to come off the medication. Each time I tried I felt terrible. I was doing all the things I recommend to patients, such as sleeping, exercising, counseling, journaling, personal time, UV light therapy and plugging in to my support community and spiritual group, but I still couldn't get off the antidepressant. It was so discouraging.

A couple of years later a friend asked me to look at the clinical research behind a supplement, which intrigued me since most supplements don't have clinical trials. I got excited after reading the studies since the supplement was formulated to improve energy levels using only three non-stimulating ingredients. At the time I wasn't sleeping more than a few hours at a time, thanks to my baby, and I was also working full time. I was exhausted and for the first time was willing to try a supplement for energy as well as a high quality vitamin supplement. Within three weeks even my husband noticed a difference in my energy level, mostly because I wasn't sneaking off for naps any more. The biggest change for me, though, was that I with the multivitamin I had also given my body the ingredients it needed to make more serotonin, and suddenly my mood started to lift. I became hopeful and slowly weaned off my antidepressant. That was years ago and I haven't needed medications since. Not only that, but I don't struggle with the anxiety and depression nearly as much as I used to, despite the ups and downs of life. It has become quite clear to me that quality supplements are an important natural remedy for depression.

MULTIVITAMINS

Everywhere you look, you are bombarded with suggestions about the next greatest thing for weight, energy, hormones, and mood. There is a bewildering array of vitamin options in every store, and watch Dr. Oz for just a few days and you'll be amazed at all the different supplements you hear about. Unfortunately many people feel they need to take all of them, and become caught up in trying to add every "latest and greatest" to their regimen. There are thousands of different over-the-counter remedies out there, and knowing which one is right for your needs is challenging. Up until just recently, the Food and Drug Administration wasn't regulating supplements the way that they monitor prescription drugs. This meant that someone could potentially mulch their lawn and put it in a capsule and call it whatever they wanted. Fortunately that has changed in the last year or so, and you can have a bit more confidence in what you are purchasing— but there are still varying degrees of quality, just like with anything in life. Good supplements have always had independent laboratory evaluations and expiration dates, but even then, finding the best one for you is the challenge. You want to make sure of a few things with your supplements. Is it safe? Is it absorbed? Is it effective?

There are a couple of different ways to know. With a high quality supplement you can start noticing differences in your physical and mental health within a few weeks. You can also ask your family or naturopathic doctor about vitamin levels. I personally use a non-invasive screening tool[3] in my office to monitor antioxidant levels, but a blood test can check on the most common vitamin levels if there is a question of whether or not your supplement is working.

I realize I haven't come out with a blanket multivitamin recommendation for everyone. I wouldn't presume to tell you which supplement brands to take, but I would say do your research and consult with your health care professional about choosing a vitamin supplement. Another great resource is a local health food store. I find their selections usually include high quality multivitamins, which I trust far more than the usual inexpensive brands found at the bigger stores.

Next I'm going to quickly cover a few other supplements that I have found to play crucial roles in helping our brains on the physical end of combating depression. I won't include dosages here, but check out the quick guide index at the end of the book for that information. Remember that supplements don't have the same regulation by the FDA that prescription medications do, which means that although they are natural, there is no guarantee they are safe or effective. I have personally used or researched several different brands over the years. I will not attempt to make a brand recommendation for all of your supplements, but I would recommend talking to a knowledgeable clerk at a private health food store if your physician doesn't have specific brand recommendations for the following supplements.

---

3. Information about this tool available at https://www.nuskin.com/en_US/products/pharmanex/scanner.html

VITAMINS D AND B

Sometimes you just need some fine-tuning. Many of us have low Vitamin D, which plays a big part in mood, bone health and energy. More and more practitioners are routinely screening for vitamin D deficiency, especially in people with celiac sprue and other medical conditions that affect absorption or bone metabolism. Recently I was feeling a bit more tired than usual and sure enough, my Vitamin D was low at 22, with the optimal level being around 50. I started 5,000 units a day and within a few days I was feeling so much better. If you are wondering if Vitamin D is a good supplement for you to take, either ask for a blood test or try 1,000 units a day, which I personally think everyone should take. You may find that you have more energy along with a slight lift in your mood.

Vitamin B6 is one of the ingredients in serotonin production, so of course it has some mood stabilizing properties. It's great for anxiety, PMS and depression, and you may notice a difference after starting 50mg a day even if your blood levels are technically normal. Most blood levels have a "normal" range but what may be normal for one person may be low for your body. So go ahead and try it. You can even try a B6/methylated folate supplement together to maximize the effects of both.

GABA, L-THEANINE AND L-GLUTAMINE

GABA is a neurotransmitter that helps calm the brain and prevent overexcitement. It is sold as a single supplement or included in mood remedies, however GABA doesn't actually cross the blood–brain barrier. So what is the blood–brain barrier? Just think of it this way: Imagine you want to get backstage at a concert, but just because you are a ticketed guest doesn't mean you have access to restricted areas. You have to have a backstage pass added to your ticket to get back there. There are bouncers that keep you out of the backstage area unless you have the pass. Your brain has its own bouncer in the form of the blood–brain barrier. So chemicals that don't get past the blood–brain barrier aren't going to have much effect on our mood, although I have had patients in the past report some improvement in their symptoms with GABA. A way around this blood–brain barrier issue is to take the main ingredients, or precursors, to the chemical we want more of in our brains. For instance, L-glutamine is a precursor to GABA and it does cross the blood–brain barrier. It's possible to get benefits from L-glutamine where there weren't any while taking GABA itself. The theory is the L-glutamine crosses into the brain and the brain then uses it to make more GABA, which then calms the brain.

Another precursor to GABA that crosses the blood–brain barrier is L-theanine. I have had fantastic results using this supplement for anxiety, both for myself and with patients. I first saw the benefits of L-theanine personally when I started taking a supplement to lower the levels of the stress hormone cortisol. One of the main ingredients was L-theanine, and within days my stress level dropped and I was able to think clearer and fall asleep easier. My second exposure to L-theanine was with a darling young patient of mine whose anxiety and depression I couldn't seem to get under control. She had failed all the usual non-prescription measures and had a strong family history of anxiety. I started her on an appropriate SSRI and she still was feeling very anxious, especially since she was heading off to college. I consulted with a psychiatrist who recommended L-theanine. It was gratifying to see her anxiety come down a tolerable level. It is not nearly as powerful a tranquilizer as ativan or xanax, but it is a good place to start and doesn't have the side effects and addiction potential of those prescription medications.

5HTP

Have you noticed yet that most of the neurotransmitters' names are bit of an alphabet soup? Well, to continue in the same vein, 5HTP is the next supplement that I find invaluable. This is frequently my first line for people who can't sleep or are feeling down. It would be great if we could just take a pill of serotonin and get our levels back up. Unfortunately it doesn't cross the blood–brain barrier—remember the bouncers that prevent access to backstage at a concert? Our brain has the equivalent and it doesn't let certain chemicals into the brain, even if they live in the brain normally. It's because there is a fine balance of serotonin needed outside of the brain also. This is why we can't just take a serotonin pill, but rather have to give the brain what it needs to make its own serotonin. There is something that does cross the blood–brain barrier, however, that can be turned into serotonin. The basic building block our brain uses to start the serotonin recipe is called 5HTP. It's related to tryptophan, which is famous for being the substance in turkey meat that makes us sleepy. I find 5HTP very helpful not only for mood stabilization but also for sleep. Just last month, for instance, I had a woman in my office who had just lost her mother, had her household income cut in half because her husband lost his job, and she herself was having some hormone changes leading up to menopause. Not surprisingly, she wasn't sleeping well. I could have tried to fiddle with her hormones but I started her on 5HTP at bedtime and within a couple of weeks she was sleeping better and feeling less stressed. I also saw a moderately depressed fifteen-year-old in the office the other day who wasn't sleeping well. We talked about exercise, light therapy, sleep hygiene, counseling and nutrition. After reviewing options with her and her mom, she chose to start 5HTP as her "medication" option. It will help her sleep, boost her mood and is much safer than prescription medications, especially at her age.

METHYLATED FOLIC ACID/L-METHYL FOLATE

I also want you to be aware of methylated folate. As we already covered, some people cannot convert regular folate to the L-methyl folate our brain uses for serotonin production, which means we lack a key ingredient and our serotonin production is severely impaired. It would be like trying to make cookies without salt. The process might be going on but the outcome is less than ideal. This means that if a person has the gene mutation that prevents that "hitching" that converts folate to methylated folate, they will never feel really well emotionally, even if they are on prescription medications to boost serotonin levels. I had a patient who was chronically depressed for years, seeing a psychiatrist, had tried multiple meds among other treatment modalities. She just never felt like she could get out from under a big black cloud. Finally we tested her for the MTHFR gene mutation. She tested positive, and we put her on L-methyl folate and within 2 weeks she felt so much better—better than she had felt in years.

INOSITOL

Are you someone who has been on meds for years and feel like they have just stopped working? Or are you someone who has tried multiple medications that worked at first but stopped working after a couple of months? Sometimes the problem isn't that we don't have enough serotonin, but rather that our bodies aren't responding to it like they should. Serotonin and dopamine transmit chemical messages, but then inside the brain cells we need a secondary messenger to finish relaying the message. That secondary messenger is inositol. It allows the serotonin to make changes to the cells in our brain. For this reason, inositol often helps with mood quickly—think of it as increasing our brains' sensitivity to the serotonin already present. It also helps people who feel like their long-term medication regimen isn't working.

ST. JOHN'S WORT

Before I end this section on supplements for mood, I would like to touch on St. John's Wort. No, it is not named after a skin infection that causes bumps all over your hands and feet. Rather "wort" is an old

English word for plant. This flowering plant has been used for centuries, beginning in ancient Greece. There have been several studies on this supplement, some of which show it to be nearly as effective as prescription-strength anti-depressants. It's not known exactly how it works in the brain but it probably works similarly to prescription pharmaceuticals, but happily does not cause decreased sex drive as most of them do. It's one of the most common over-the-counter supplements purchased in the United States. Sounds fantastic, right? The only thing you need to be aware of is that because it is powerful, it can have side effects. Just like the prescription drugs, it can cause nausea, fatigue, upset stomach, and headaches. Most of those side effects will improve with continued use, but it can also cause a light sensitivity rash which will only get worse with repeated sun exposure. Even more concerning, it can interfere with many different medications as well as the liver's ability to process chemicals. Certain heart prescriptions, blood thinners, anesthesia drugs and birth control are all less effective when taking St. John's Wort, just to name a few. There is a long list of possible interactions so please consult your physician if you are thinking of starting this supplement and are already taking a prescription. If you are not on any other medications or supplements then this is an effective over-the-counter option that most likely acts like a stopper for the sink in your brain, leading to increased levels of serotonin over a few weeks time.

Aside from the St. John's Wort, all the supplements we reviewed in this chapter are safe for you to try on your own. Allow 3–4 weeks on a supplement before you give up on it, and make sure to take it regularly. If you are someone who forgets to take your medications or supplements, try putting them by your toothbrush or putting a reminder on your phone. The trick is not to turn it off until you take the medication—don't swipe the timer until you swallow the pill!

Chapter 3
Other Ways of Boosting Your Serotonin Levels

Swallowing a pill, powder or liquid isn't the only way to boost the serotonin levels in our brain. Let's cover a few basic things you can do to help balance the chemicals in your brain. First let me say that I know this list may seem overwhelming when you are weighed down with depression, so please don't feel you need to do all of these things. Just start with one thing at a time.

SUNLIGHT

Yes, the full UV spectrum available in sunlight is very good for our brains, boosting our levels of serotonin. A wonderful article in 2007 explained that we get far less sunlight daily than our ancestors. Because we spend the majority of our lives inside, rather than outside hunting, gathering or farming, we tend to get far less light than our brains were genetically programmed to want and need. Even on a cloudy day we get several times more light outside than we do inside. Of course we don't go around testing brain levels of serotonin in living humans so we don't have a direct measurement of how much light is needed to raise the levels in your brain, but we know for sure there is a link. When serotonin levels were measured in brains during autopsy, the levels of serotonin were higher in the summer than in the winter.[4]

---

4. Simon N. Young, "How to Increase Serotonin in the Human Brain Without Drugs." J Psychiatry Neuroscience, 2007 Nov: 32(6): 394-399

So what does this all mean for you? It means that more sunlight is better, although my dermatologist would disagree. To that point, it's less about the sunlight on our skin than it is full spectrum UV light activating the retina. Yes, it would be great to get outside in bright light for twenty-five minutes a day, but we can easily accomplish the same effect with a full spectrum UV light. There are a variety of light therapy devices on the market ranging in price from $15 for one full-spectrum UV lightbulb in the plant section of your local superstore, or you can get on amazon.com and find a variety of light boxes from $36 to $300. If it is a light box or bulb that you are using, then you want to put it facing your eyes at an angle so you can read facing the light or get ready for the day in front of it so the UV rays shine into your eyes. If you are not likely to be stationary for 20-25 minutes, there are also wearable options in the form of hats with lights built into the brims. Whatever form you choose, light therapy is remarkably effective and safe for everyone from children to pregnant women to the elderly. It is also a first line therapy for those suffering from Seasonal Affective Disorder, which is a term for the major mood changes some people experience during the winter months that have shorter sunlight hours. Whatever your situation, light therapy is a great place to start.

EXERCISE

Now, I know that for some this is a dirty word, and for others it conjures up images of sweaty, grunting muscle-heads at the gym. I want you to put all that aside for a moment. What if I had the magic pill that could help you feel more relaxed, help you lose weight and gain muscle, help prevent strokes and heart attacks, help you sleep better, improve your libido and help you think more clearly? What would you be willing to pay for that kind of supplement? If I could come up with that magical pill, I'd be a billionaire and win the Nobel Prize all in one year. Unfortunately there is no pill, there is only you moving your body.

Don't call it exercise if that word freaks you out, and don't go out and start a new routine that isn't enjoyable for you. The most effective exercise you can do is what you are already doing. If you walk, step up the speed or frequency. If you like to dance then dance, whether it's in your living room, a zumba class or following a YouTube video. If you like to garden then do it briskly and for a minimum of fifteen minutes. It takes only fifteen to twenty minutes of some form of movement that makes you sweat and breathe quickly, as little as four days a week, to make a difference in how you are feeling physically, mentally and emotionally. Whether that is hauling rocks, shooting hoops, riding a bike, dancing, yoga, sex, raking the lawn, scrubbing floors, or running, it all counts as exercise. The physical activity you do will give you all the benefits I listed above, plus there is an added benefit of an endorphin "high." Endorphins are chemicals produced in our brains that act a bit like morphine, both suppressing pain and giving a feeling of euphoria, and they are often released during exercise. You will hear people talk about a runner's high, which is the very natural and pleasant euphoria from endorphin release and it's a great mood booster. So clearly there are many benefits to exercise and hopefully one will motivate you to add more movement to your daily routine.

I'll share a story, since that is always more interesting than just reading a list of things to try. I self medicated my depression with exercise from the time I was eleven and learned to ride horses. If I could get outside and do something physical at least four days a week, I was a happy and relaxed girl. If I couldn't, then I was anxious and moody and snappy with my brothers and sisters. When we moved from a small town to a big city and I couldn't ride my horse anymore, I began playing softball and basketball and volleyball. After high school I took aerobic exercise classes in college, but only sporadically, and then wondered why some semesters I was tired and anxious all the time. Of course it was the semesters I didn't have an exercise class three days a week that I was struggling with my energy and mood. I finally made the connection in medical school and started running. At first it was a painful trot alternating with fast walking, but then I worked up to three to five miles at a time and my energy and mood were fantastic, even during the stress of med school. I continued to run for fifteen years as my primary form of exercise.

I thought that was all I needed, but in residency I developed daily headaches at the base of my skull for six months. They were brutal, and nothing I did touched them: ibuprofen, Tylenol, running, massage therapy, and chiropractic visits all failed to give me relief. Only sleeping helped and that wasn't something I could rely on since I was working 100 hours a week and up frequently at night. One day, on a whim, I bought the AM/PM Yoga DVD from Gaiam. It was a simple fifteen-minute yoga routine for beginners that I could do either morning or night. Within four days my headaches were gone. Even to this day, if I get a tension headache and do fifteen minutes of yoga, all is well. Before you start imagining me as some flexible yogi master, please know that I can barely touch my toes and have only been to a yoga studio a few times in my life. I am a closet and casual yoga practitioner, but even that brings me great benefits, both physically and mentally. I am definitely more relaxed and focused on the days I do yoga.

As a contrast to the above story about the benefits of exercise, I learned the hard way how horrible it is when I don't exercise. My last two pregnancies were during my late thirties, and my obstetrician put me on exercise restriction due to premature contractions. Unlike my first pregnancy, when I ran up until the last two weeks, I couldn't even walk briskly the second half of my last two pregnancies. Let me tell you, I was a wreck. I was tearful and anxious and moody far beyond normal hormonal shifts, and I also developed major digestive issues and fatigue that were debilitating. The only thing that kept me functional during those pregnancies was weekly acupuncture, which I was able to quit the minute I started exercising again.

Just this last fall I was again reminded how important exercise is to my mental health. I was diagnosed with early arthritis in my hip and the orthopedist told me that I either quit running now or I was looking at a hip replacement before I was fifty. At that point I didn't know of any other way to get an endorphin high in twenty minutes. Running was the most convenient and fastest way to get all the benefits from exercise. I struggled for about two months to get in a good workout that boosted my mood and didn't hurt my hip and didn't take an hour from door to door. My mood slowly spiraled downward during that time, and I was definitely struggling with depression as the winter months approached. Thankfully, I was stuck at home one day and, feeling crazy, I searched for "home cardio workouts, no equipment" and up popped a free website that has changed my life: fitnessblender. com. I will forever be grateful to that couple who have put together beautiful, fun, easy-to-follow workouts that anyone can do at home.

Clearly for me, exercise has been part of my life for over thirty years, but I know that exercise is daunting for most people. Often people struggle with making this a habit and don't know where to start. If you are currently doing nothing but walking from your car to your office and back to your car, start by parking as far from your office as you can. Often we pride ourselves on finding the prime parking spots, as if it's a sign of cosmic good luck or brilliant strategizing on our part if we can park as close to the entrance as possible. Instead, make the choice to do yourself a favor and park as far from the entrance as you can, whether it's your office or the grocery store or the library or where ever you go regularly. It honestly doesn't take much physical movement to make a difference in your emotional and physical health. If you can move for fifteen minutes a day, four days a week you will see a difference. Preferably it will be movement that makes you breathe hard and sweat, but even walking across the parking lot is a place to start.

Some people have very physical jobs and come home exhausted at the end of the day. Physically demanding work is not the same as exercise—it doesn't tend to give you the mental relaxation that planned exercise does, so try to add something to your routine that you enjoy and that helps you relax.

There are also those on the opposite end of the spectrum who truly have physical restrictions, bad joints, etc. To you I suggest checking out Sit and Be Fit YouTube videos. I did some of these when I was pregnant and they can really make you sweat! Basically they are workouts you can do sitting down and are wonderful for elderly, pregnant women, arthritic patients or anyone with weight bearing restrictions.

If you are thinking that you never have fifteen minute time slots to exercise, don't use it as an excuse to not start at all. Even three sessions of brisk exercise lasting five minutes each instead of a single fifteen minute session will help with weight loss and cardiovascular health. There will not likely be an endorphin high, but you will still have the satisfaction of completing your exercise goal and taking charge of your health.

Obviously I could go on and on about the importance of exercise, but I will just sum it up this way. Everyone will benefit in some way from exercise, so start moving today!

SLEEP

I cannot emphasize enough how important sleep is. It is the time our body uses to restore and repair itself, to produce more of its necessary hormones and neurotransmitters, and much detoxification takes place while we are sleeping. Sleep also renews our energy and allows us to function optimally.

Too many of us don't get enough sleep. I'm not going to tell you that you need eight hours of sleep, because many people need far less than that, but I will say that we should be getting enough sleep that we feel restored in the morning. Unfortunately there is a tendency to burn the candle at both ends by staying up very late and getting up early. My question is always, why are you up so late? The most common response I hear is "That's the only time I have to myself." We are all busy; our days are consumed with work, housework, errands, kids, volunteering, appointments, phone calls, social media, the list goes on and on. By the end of the day our energy is low, so we tend to check out after dinner and relax. It could be watching TV for hours or disappearing into social media, and too often a short "break" turns into hours and suddenly it's late at night and we have cut into our sleep time. Not just that, but we frequently also have a hard time falling asleep after a crazy day of stress without exercise, and we think that relaxing in front of the TV or computer will help us fall asleep. Unfortunately anything with a backlight, meaning anything that shines a light in your eyes, actually keeps you awake.

The point I'm making is that we need to plan ahead and make sure we are getting to bed before too late so we can get excellent restorative sleep, which includes REM sleep and dreaming. If you are guilty of staying up too late and waking up exhausted the next morning, set an alarm an hour before you want to be asleep so you will be reminded to start your bedtime routine earlier. If you are someone who has problems falling asleep, turn off your backlit electronics an hour before bed and let your brain wind down with music or journaling or a bath or meditation. If you are someone who wakes up in the middle of the night and cannot get back to sleep, please don't turn on all the lights or the TV. Read a boring book by lamplight instead.

Clearly there are many people with actual sleep disorders who have far greater challenges than just a few poor sleep habits. Low serotonin affects sleep, and the classic early sign of depression is awakening around two or three a.m. and having difficulty getting back to sleep. It's one of the first symptoms to appear and the last to get better as your serotonin levels go back up. The 5HTP at bedtime will help with this a bit, as will the exercise, but the process is slow so don't be too anxious if you aren't sleeping through the night. If you are awake longer than twenty minutes, then get up and have a cup of warm herbal tea and relax for a minute with a non-stimulating book and then try going back to bed. It will get better.

Menopause is another time when sleep is greatly disrupted due to the drop in hormone levels. Depending upon the severity of your sleep problems it may be worth seeing a healthcare professional about your options. Chronic insomniacs don't need me to tell them about sleep difficulties, but I will just say that if you have had problems falling or staying asleep since you were a child and haven't seen a health care provider, please do so. There are various options open to you, not all of which have to be prescription drugs. I frequently use 5HTP, melatonin, L-theanine, valerian root, and even Benadryl or Unisom with my patients who have mild to moderate sleep problems. Again, I would suggest seeing your own doctor to fine tune your regimen, but usually these over-the-counter supplements and remedies are a safe place to start.

The last caveat I will bring up is Obstructive Sleep Apnea. This is a medical condition where people have pauses in their breathing which causes oxygen levels to drop. This leads to a whole host of problems, including hypertension, type 2 diabetes, low testosterone, poor concentration and extreme tiredness. People with sleep apnea are often overweight or obese, usually snore significantly, and if observed will have pauses in their snoring and breathing. They wake up feeling like a wreck, as if they haven't slept, because the dips in oxygen will severely disrupt their sleep cycle and bring them partially if not fully awake. People with sleep apnea frequently struggle with staying awake during the day and I often hear them complain that it's impossible to lose weight. If this picture sounds familiar to you, please talk to your doctor about it, because no amount of sleep medication will ever help you sleep well until you are treated for your obstructive sleep apnea.

On the whole, setting aside medical conditions that cause sleep issues, the majority of people who aren't getting enough sleep are just staying up too late at night doing unimportant things that I call "brain dead fun." Candy Crush, Facebook and Twitter, TV and Netflix all fall into that category. Those are all fine in moderation but don't get sucked so far in that you are losing chunks of your sleeping time, or other important parts of your life to these escapes. If you feel you need them to relax, again, use them in moderation—or better yet, do ten minutes of yoga or some other exercise and see how you sleep. We all know we feel better when we go to bed at a reasonable hour and get enough sleep. So just do it!

MEDICAL CARE

As I mentioned before, this book and the suggestions here are not supposed to replace medical care, especially if you are suffering from severe depression or other mood disorders such as bipolar disorder or schizophrenia. Severe depression is dangerous, and if you are having thoughts of suicide or harming yourself, it's an emergency situation, just as important as any other medical emergency such as chest pain or extremely high blood sugars. Too often we feel "it's only in my head." You are right in that the chemical imbalances are all in your brain, but it is as real a condition as diabetes, hypertension or emphysema. Please don't ignore it.

Some people have such severe depression that they don't respond well to anti-depressant medication, mood stabilizers or counseling. For those cases there is a relatively new treatment modality available in some places, called Transcranial Magnetic Stimulation. Basically it's a big magnet that is targeted to stimulate parts of the brain such as the prefrontal cortex that are underactive in people with severe depression. It's safe and non-invasive and is definitely worth looking into if other options have failed.

It is always important to consider professional medical care with severe depression, but it's critical to consider when there is any degree of depression in pregnant women, post partum women, teenagers, or anyone with thoughts of suicide. If you or your loved one falls into that category I would strongly suggest making an appointment with a health care professional immediately to discuss options. It isn't just that you need to be evaluated for the severity of your depression and the need for medication; it's also about being plugged into a support system which includes a doctor as well as a counselor. Counseling alone is as effective as medication in treating mild to moderate depression. Pregnant women and nursing moms will need guidance about which supplements or medications are safe to use, and teenagers are their own special group.

PART 2
MENTAL

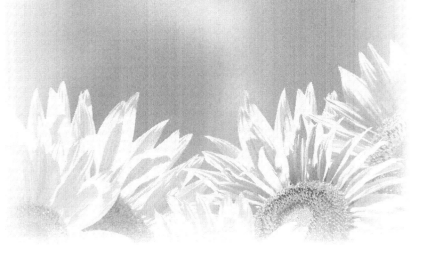

Chapter 4
What Are You Thinking?

In the last section we talked about the physical and chemical changes that lead to depression and anxiety. If it were as simple as changing the physical condition of a patient through medication then we would have eradicated most diseases ages ago. Of course it's not that simple because there is always the equally powerful influence of our mind and spirit on our mood disorders. I want to talk about the power of our thoughts, both conscious and subconscious. They are incredibly powerful, just as powerful as brain chemistry—or in my opinion even more so. I will share my personal experience in this arena and you can relate it to your situation.

THE POWER OF OUR THOUGHTS

Our thoughts have power, which is becoming more accepted since it has been scientifically proven. This concept is even being utilized in the commercial gaming industry: the company NeuroSky has developed a headset that allows users to control a game with only their thoughts. If we can control things outside of our body with just our thoughts, clearly we can change the state of our bodies with the thoughts that we think. I will talk more about this later on the book, but I bring it up now to make the point that our thoughts are arguably as powerful as the chemicals in our brain. That being said, what are you thinking?

I was in medical school when the movie Patch Adams came out. I had just learned about serotonin and the delicate balance of neurotransmitters in the brain and how depression is a physical condition, not just an attitude like many people believe. I heard my professor say that Patch Adams in essence felt depression was just loneliness and if we were better friends to each other we could get rid of depression. I thought, "He clearly doesn't understand the neurochemistry of depression." I laugh at the arrogant little puppy I was. So much of depression is, of course, the circumstances we find ourselves in as well as the thoughts we think daily. Can those be changed without medication? Absolutely.

If you had known my views fifteen years ago you would realize this is a radical shift for me. I always believed that you could make things happen in your life with hard work and willpower. I had no doubts that I would get into medical school because every morning I read my goal to myself out loud. "I, Raphael Montana Allred, will start medical school at the University of Utah in September 1994." I firmly believe that my posture and confidence going into my interviews stemmed from the belief I had planted in my subconscious with that affirmation.

Despite that experience, I had the view that when it comes to matters of health, we have no control over what we inherit from our parents, and that my depression was something I would always struggle with because it was hereditary. I had the same view about the chronic inflammatory conditions in my family. I felt I had no control over the fibromyalgia, just as I had no control over the depression, because they were both hereditary. I have an uncle on my father's side who committed suicide, a great uncle on my mother's side who committed suicide, and I watched my dad struggle with depression for as long as I can remember. In my mind, it was just how it was. I felt helpless and that the only hope came from the fact that we now have really good medications compared with fifty years ago.

I first started on prescription medication for depression during my first year in practice. I had made it through the stress of medical school and residency without medication despite the anxiety and intermittent depression. Looking back I realize it's because I had a fantastic support system in both places, as well as a clear goal I was working toward. Once I started into practice, however, I had suddenly "arrived" and wasn't working toward any exciting goals anymore. It was a big transition time, including buying my first house and moving far away from my birth family, as well as getting engaged. Of course these changes were all positive, but I found them overwhelming and became depressed. I tried a couple of different medications, and despite being on an SSRI, I ended up on a second medication after I got married and was struggling with that adjustment. My sweet husband, although supportive, had a totally different view of depression and anxiety. He expressed to me the belief that we have control over our health and that I had the power to change it. I became very defensive and angry and said, "You don't understand! You've never been depressed and no one in your family suffers from depression."

Let me pause here for a moment and take a look at my attitude. For one thing, I was still living with the beliefs I had grown up with: that our family just had poor health, and that depression ran in our family. I was also living with the belief that depression is chemical and therefore I had no control over it. Underlying all of that was the subconscious fear of taking control of my life. I was comfortable being a victim of my genetics and physical health, because then I wasn't responsible for my ultimate success or failure. I had an excuse if I didn't progress in life or even make an effort. I had assumed the role of a sick person, to a certain extent, and it was both my burden and my security. This is a critical point I want to make: Are you hiding behind your depression on a subconscious level? Are there any rewards in being a depressed or anxious person, such as extra attention or special consideration from others? Are you willing to leave the sick role behind and choose to do everything in your power to be well? It's a very scary thought, because suddenly there is the risk of failure— what if you don't achieve absolute wellness and still struggle, and are disappointed in the outcome? It's also scary because suddenly you have to take responsibility for yourself. It's so much easier to blame our circumstances for our life, health or bad luck than it is to say, "Today I chose to take control of my life and whatever happens will be up to me." Yes, there are people who experience horrible tragedy out of their control, but how they react is always within their control. It comes down to one question—do you want to be a depressed person or do you want to be a happy person who occasionally feels down?

"STOP IT"

I was certainly not ready to let go of my identity as a depressed and anxious person during the first couple of years of my marriage. I would resist and feel resentful if my husband ever suggested I had the ability to change my emotional and mental state. We managed to inject some humor into the subject shortly after my first baby was born and I began having panic attacks. He had seen a Saturday Night Live skit where Bob Newhart played a psychiatrist who only charged $5 for his sessions because he had a one sentence treatment that he used for everything. The "patient" explained that she had a terrible fear of being buried alive, and further had developed claustrophobia to the point that she didn't even want to go into a building. Bob then leaned over the desk and told her he was going to give her two words that would be all she needed to change everything. He then proceeded to shout, "STOP IT!" As if that would fix everything and she should just decide to stop it when she felt claustrophobic or thought about being buried alive. It's hilarious of course because it's so ridiculous. Or is it? Clearly you can't stop a phobia overnight, but what about how you perceive the phobia, the depression, the anxiety?

I was in the middle of a panic attack one night and I said to my husband, "I can't breathe. I feel like my chest is squeezing the air off!" Looking back I'm sure he was feeling a bit overwhelmed between the screaming baby and the panicking wife, but he gave me a little smile and said, "Well, just stop it." I gave a little giggle because it was so ridiculous but it actually helped. Over the next five years as we had two more children and I continued to struggle with my depression and go on and off meds, his go-to response whenever I would complain of feeling that way was, "Just stop it." He said it in a humorous way but on some level he was serious about wanting me to take control of my life and change how I was responding to my circumstances. The question was whether or not I really, on a subconscious as well as conscious level, wanted to let go of my identity as a depressed and anxious person.

Chapter 5
Choosing to Be Happy

I used to feel so irritated when people would say, "Happiness is a choice." I felt they didn't understand what I was going through or that they had never been depressed. What I didn't understand is that we don't always get to choose the circumstances in our lives, but we do get to choose how we react to them.

Let me use an analogy. Let's talk about weight. There are fat people and skinny people and a lot of in between people. Some of us are born to families that have chronic obesity and our weight is always a chronic struggle. Some families have high metabolism and can eat whatever they want and never gain any weight, or only have to exercise to keep it under control. But there are some families that have super low metabolism and hang onto every calorie. Is it fair that you just look at ice cream and gain weight? No, it's not. But as we know, life isn't fair. That's just how it is and we have the choice of saying, "Well, obesity runs in my family, that's just how I will end up," or we can say, "I know I'm predisposed to obesity but I will do everything in my power not to become obese. I may not be super-skinny but I won't end up with obesity-related health issues that control my life."

It's the same thing with depression and anxiety. We can say, "I am depressed and anxious because it's genetic," or even, "I'm depressed because I've had trauma or a hard life." The alternative is to say, "I have been dealt a hand that I don't like, and I struggle with feeling anxious or depressed, but I'm going to be in control of how I react and

I will do everything I can not to focus on the depression. I choose to be happy!" Will you always feel happy? No, of course not. Just like a person who struggles with obesity won't always lose weight even though he is trying. But you can have the intention to always try.

It takes more than just intention, of course. Otherwise we would all be skinny and rich because that's what we intended when we were younger. The real key is to find tools that work for you—tools that help put your focus on positive thoughts which will combat depression. Let's explore a few of those tools.

FUEL YOUR BRAIN

Clearly the literal nutritional fuel for our brain is important but I also want to talk about what we fuel our brain with intellectually. There are always the physical, mental and emotional sides of things and I will talk later about the emotional and spiritual aspect of our brain health. I also talked earlier about the physical aspects of mental health. I want to talk about third component to mental health, which is the thoughts that we put into our brains. Just as you fuel your brain with food, you also fuel your brain with images, sounds and thoughts every moment of every day. Sometimes we take out old memories and run them like a movie reel. Sometimes we escape into actual movies or TV or video games. Other times we listen to music or have conversations. Even if you don't consciously choose to fill your brain, it is going to happen and unfortunately people too often choose the default of not making a decision and letting life just happen to them, of fueling their brain with anything and everything that they encounter along the way. Too often we fail to realize the impact of our "fuel" choices on our mood.

Let's talk specifics. Let's look at the movies, books, music and conversations that you surround yourself with daily. Do they leave you feeling uplifted and happy or do they leave you feeling depressed, restless, anxious, bored or in some other negative state of mind? Are you focusing on all the bad news in the world and watching the violent or disturbing footage over and over? Are you engaging in frustrating political or religious debates?

I'm not judging your choices—I'm just asking you to notice the cost to your emotional and mental state of being. I find it interesting that when I am feeling depressed I am drawn to depressing news and entertainment. For years I would watch scary or angry shows, read fiction that left me feeling irritable and restless, and listen to music that was far from soothing or uplifting. I fight that tendency now, but in the past I found it masochistically satisfying on some level to punish myself with more fuel for self-destruction. Once I consciously recognized what I was doing I chose to stop that cycle and reach for uplifting movies, music and books instead. Do another experiment for five days— deliberately choose uplifting books and movies and conversations and see what your mood does.

SELF TALK

The other area of fuel for our brain is the self-talk we use. What are we telling our brain, our subconscious? There is a great book by Shad Helmstetter, *What to Say When you Talk To Yourself*, that uncovers what we are really saying to ourselves and how to deprogram those negative thoughts. Our mind is our most powerful organ in our body, and whatever it believes is true, will become so in our physical health. I remember hearing the story about the man who froze to death on the train when he got locked in a refrigeration box car. He wrote of his despair and how cold he felt the hours before he died. The irony is that the box car wasn't hooked up to power and the temperature was only slightly less than the outside summer night air. His brain told his body he was going to die, so he did.

Clearly that is an extreme example, but my question to you is, what is your brain telling your body? We will talk more about this later, but basically, your brain is saying whatever you tell it to say. This is where affirmations come in. Think of an affirmation as an "I will…" statement that lets your brain know what positive thing you are planning on doing and seeing in the near future so it can work with you.

I used an affirmation when applying to medical school, and then promptly forgot about them for years. I was very happily reminded of affirmations when I read the life-changing book *Miracle Morning*, by Hal Elrod. That book played a huge part in the shift in my mentality, my belief and my energy level. Writing this book was a direct result of reading that book. I began fueling my mind with affirmations morning and night for weeks and months. I was telling myself what I was planning on doing the next day, how I would feel when I woke up and how each day was precious to my life. I told myself what I would accomplish in all areas of my life. You can create an affirmation about anything. Napoleon Hill was a great believer in the power of thoughts and he has a sample affirmation in his classic, *Think and Grow Rich*. Hal Elrod also has wonderful resources on his website for *Miracle Morning*, including sample affirmations. The key to a powerful affirmation is knowing what you want in life.

HAVING A GOAL

Knowing what you want isn't as simple as it sounds. Sure, who doesn't want to be financially secure and healthy and happy? But what does happiness look like? Too often we equate happiness with a tangible object, location, achievement or circumstance in life. I used to think, "I will be happy when…." I was waiting for something wonderful to happen before I would allow myself to be happy. But spectacular events are not what true happiness is about, of course. As Roy M. Goodman said, "Happiness is a way of travel—not a destination."

One of my favorite wake-up calls about happiness came while reading The *Hidden Messages in Water* by Dr. Emoto Masaru. He simply asks, "Do you have a sense of peace in your heart, a feeling of security about your future, and a feeling of anticipation when you wake up in the morning?

If we can call this happiness, then would you say that at this moment you are happy?" Most people would say no, because peace, security and anticipation can be elusive. It's the anticipation I want to focus on for a moment. Anticipation implies that you are waiting for something good to happen. Pooh Bear so eloquently describes the excitement of anticipation as that moment before eating the honey that is better than actually eating the honey. If we apply this to having a goal, part of happiness is the anticipation of reaching the destination, the excitement and joy of the challenge. Clearly having a purpose is critical and for me I was at my most depressed when I wasn't working toward a goal.

So what is your goal? What we want will change depending upon the time or season of life, but unless we have a clear intention and work toward it, we will rob ourselves of the joy of anticipation. And of course, if we don't have a destination we will never reach it. Instead we will wander aimlessly, letting life decide for us because we never choose for ourselves, letting life take us places we don't like because we didn't plan for something specific.

This point was driven home to me when I read a work of fiction by author Andy Andrews. In *The Traveler's Gift* the main character is in despair, with his life in ruins around him. His "gift" is to travel through time to meet some of history's greatest leaders. While visiting with one of them he is told that his current circumstances are a result of the decisions and choices he has made up to that point. He, of course, violently rejects this notion. Who would want to take accountability for a life that is in ruins? I didn't like that thought any more than the fictional character did.

Around the same time, though, I took a course titled "Call to Action" from brilliant life coach, Michael Bernoff. The course helped me take a good look at my life, highlighting the areas lacking progress and the reasons why I wasn't progressing. I was given fantastic tools, and in the end I re-examined the choices that I make daily and yearly and realized something disturbing. I wasn't making choices. I was just getting up, going through the routine of life and not working toward anything. I wasn't living life, I was letting life happen to me.

At that point I started making goals again, and having just read *Miracle Morning* I started using the power of affirmations to keep myself focused on my destination. I made goals for my physical health, for my marriage, for my income level and my personal development. I started exploring new business ventures that brought passion and excitement back into my life. I suddenly felt more alive than I had in years. Everyone needs a purpose.

If you are still not clear on what you really want to do or be in life—or even if you are—I would highly recommend *You are a Badass* by Jen Sincero. Not only is the book highly entertaining, but it powerfully and concisely summarizes the struggles we face on our journey to become our best selves, as well as explaining the tools we need to develop that will aid us in this process. It is empowering and motivating. Do yourself a favor and get the book.

LAUGHTER AND FUN

Another tool that is too often under-utilized is laughter. When was the last time you had a belly laugh? The kind of laugh that makes it hard to breathe? Unfortunately for most of us, it is rarely every day. Even a chuckle or a giggle isn't always a frequent occurrence. On the other hand, watch babies and young children. They are always laughing and giggling and half the time it's not clear why! One thing is clear, however; they are much more relaxed and happy than most adults. Why is that?

The benefits of laughter rival those of exercise. When we truly laugh, our brains release endorphins and serotonin, among other things. It's an instant feel good for our brain and our mood. For most people, spending time with friends and family results in more laughter than watching or listening to something funny, but do whatever it takes to bring more happy, hearty laughter into your life.

Along with that, have fun! I find myself getting serious as a heart attack about life sometimes. Yes, my job does deal with serious things like heart attacks, but the rest of the time there is no need to attack life with that kind of seriousness. It's tremendously important to let loose and have fun with people we love and trust. That is when we laugh. That is when we have fun and feel relaxed and happy. It can be something as simple as dancing in front of your computer with your kids, which is my favorite way of having fun regularly, or it can be a girls' or guys' night out, cosmic bowling, paintball, movies or comedy clubs. Just make sure you plan your fun if you are an innately serious person, otherwise life becomes a chore, which is a downer.

GRATITUDE

When was the last time you stopped and looked around and counted your blessings? What are the people, opportunities, privileges or comforts in your life you are grateful for? I know I forget to focus on these things when I am feeling stressed and unhappy. Ironically, focusing on my blessings and living in a space of gratitude is the best solution for stress and depression.

Too often we focus on what we don't have, which promotes feelings of dissatisfaction and unhappiness. Live in that space long enough and the unhappiness turns into depression. If instead of wallowing in what we don't have, we focus on what we already do have, we'll create feelings of gratitude. When we live in gratitude we create an energetic space in our lives that attracts more abundance, more things, people and circumstances we can be grateful for. Michael Losier does an excellent job explaining this in his book *Law of Attraction*. Basically, our thoughts are like magnifying glasses and what we focus on in life becomes larger. If we spend our time thinking about our lacks, our depression, our stress, we will attract more of that into our lives. If we instead focus on how many wonderful things we have already, such as a working brain and body, clothes, safety, political freedom, warm houses, indoor plumbing, on-line shopping, food, and friends, we will attract more wonderful things into our lives.

I found this concept to be powerful when applied to emotions in relationships. I was feeling frustrated in many of my relationships—

both at home and at work and wanted to have more joy and ease with my loved ones. A brilliant mentor of mine told me, "Whatever you water will grow. You may as well water the flowers instead of the weeds." I did an experiment with my marriage and instead of focusing on areas I wished my husband would change, I focused on his many, many positive attributes and the thoughtful ways he cares for his family. Suddenly my frustrations with my husband were almost non-existent and I felt happier in my marriage than I ever had.

We live in a world that spends a tremendous amount of energy complaining and looking at the negative side of things. When we fall into that trap we are just asking the universe for more of the same negative results. Making the shift to a place of gratitude not only attracts positive things into your life, but it also helps change your attitude and perception of events. Suddenly the little things in life aren't such a big deal and you will find your stress level dropping dramatically. So do an experiment for a week and make a list nightly of all the things you are grateful for, all the ways you have been blessed that day. You will be amazed at how quickly you will start to feel better.

JOURNALING

There is something very therapeutic in writing our thoughts, our memories, our dreams, our intentions. Like affirmations, journaling is a powerful tool to focus our thoughts and intentions. It makes us aware of patterns and ruts, fears and hesitations and most of all, the places and things we spend our mental energy on. As you take five minutes a day and record what you are thinking about and then read back over the journal, you may be surprised to discover what you think about most. Will those things be important in five years? Are you expending mental energy on improving yourself or complaining about your circumstances? It's only when we are conscious of our current thought patterns that we can begin to change them.

MAKING THE SHIFT

I have listed only a few of the tools you can use in your life, but there are thousands of resources available to you. The key is to open yourself to the possibility of change. The change can be a slow progression or it can be overnight. Over the last three years I have had a flurry of activity focused around personal development, life goals and progression. That coincided with my passionate desire to stop taking antidepressants for good. For me it was a major shift. It was a shift in my beliefs about what was possible for my health, a shift in my willingness to abandon the role of a being a depressed person, and a shift in the level of effort I was willing to put into changing my life.

When and why you arrive at this pivotal shift is different for everyone, but for me it was because I had reached an all-time low. I knew I couldn't live in that space, if only for the sake of my children. I also desperately wanted to be happy again, and if I wanted different results than I was getting, then I had to be willing to do something different than what I had been doing. If you are reading this book you are probably somewhere in that neighborhood.

Sometimes that can be a very scary space, standing on the precipice of a change. This is especially true if we have emotional baggage or trauma that has held us down in our lives. Let me just encourage you to keep going! I know you can make the changes you need to in order to be in control of your own happiness.

PART 3
EMOTIONAL

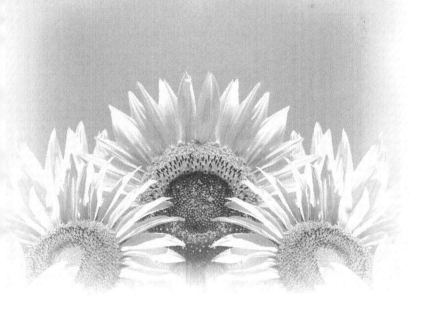

Chapter 6
Life Hurts

All of us are wounded by life. My mom was once bemoaning the fact that she had unknowingly made a mistake with one of her children that had led to problems for him as an adult. I told her, "Mom, no one gets out of childhood without baggage." If we are fortunate, it is life's ordinary disappointments such as loneliness or isolation, or the unintentional thoughtlessness of those around us that causes the hurt. Unfortunately, too many in the world experience actual trauma, either as a child or as an adult. We too often pack these hurts from life into our bags and carry them around with us, not because we want to, but because we don't know how to unpack the bags. We continue to wound ourselves daily by mentally replaying the painful experience over and over in our minds, like a bad rerun.

Clearly what is traumatic for one person is just something unfortunate for another. I find it interesting to look back at different generations. Death used to be a normal part of life up until the last century, and now we live in a time when lives are prolonged through modern medicine to the point that we struggle to handle it when we lose a loved one.

Political tyranny is also a thing that is foreign to most of us. I compare my life to those of the millions of refugees who have fled political tyranny, war or violence through the ages. Most recently the millions of refugees from the Middle East and Africa fleeing oppression have seen things that I will never have to contemplate in my life. Over half the refugees are children, which is gut-wrenching. These families have been left without possessions, without a way of feeding or clothing themselves or their children. When I think about these things I suddenly feel that my struggles are no longer a big deal.

That being said, putting my hurts into perspective doesn't eradicate the experience or the wound it left behind. A wound is a wound and it hurts. There is no explaining why something is very traumatic for one person when another person looking in wouldn't feel it's a big deal. I will tell a couple of stories to illustrate what I mean.

I had a friend who was shy and clumsy as a kid and she never felt she fit in. She was teased, and because of it she had this perception of herself as stupid and unattractive. She had terrible self esteem and this developed into terrible self-talk, which developed into self-destructive behavior. It took her years of counseling and hard work to pull herself out of that spiral. Now, on the surface, being clumsy and getting teased are clearly not the end of the world, but to her it was a huge deal and left a major emotional wound.

My family moved from Montana to Salt Lake City the summer I turned fifteen. Doesn't sound too bad, does it? My little sister, the social butterfly, was overjoyed. Bigger school, more friends and the hustle of the city sounded like heaven to her. For me, it was extremely traumatic. My love and joy in life was riding my horse through the forest and up the mountain trails. My dearest friends, as well as my grandmother, lived just through the woods from my house. It was idyllic. Leaving it behind was like ripping a hole inside of me that I didn't know how to heal. The world was gray. I lost some trust in my parents and I dreaded going to school. I slept to escape and withdrew into myself. Fortunately my fabulous parents were very present in my life and took me to see a great doctor. She educated me about depression and helped shift my perspective on what was happening, as well as encouraging me to exercise instead of taking medication.

My mom also told me a story about an elderly woman, Evelyn, who had to move in with her son and daughter-in-law because she couldn't support herself. She was cheerful and helpful with the grandkids every day, but when she finally died and her daughter-in-law read Evelyn's journal, she was shocked to find out how unhappy Evelyn had been living in someone else's home and being dependent upon them. Evelyn had just chosen to be cheerful and helpful despite her own unhappiness. My mom was a wise woman, making the point without coming out and saying it, and I realized I had been selfish and decided to become more helpful and cheerful. Life went on without my horse, without my friends and without my grandmother through the woods, and I took back my happiness.

Again, in the big scheme of things, was moving to the city really a traumatic event? No one hurt me, no one molested me or threatened me, I wasn't separated from my family and no one died. Sounds like I blew it all out of proportion, right? Well, to me it was a big deal, and I had to honor that and go through the mourning process and heal, like we all do from any trauma, big or small.

The last story I will tell relates to my youngest daughter. Again, on the surface, it wasn't a huge deal, but to me it was the single most traumatic thing I've been through. While I was pregnant I found out she had a cleft lip and palate. I knew that would mean multiple painful surgeries and I also knew it meant that she wouldn't be able to breast feed, which was one of my greatest joys with my other two children. I was devastated, for her and for me. When she was four months old she had her first surgery; it was just as horrible as I was dreading, and she actually ended up re-hospitalized with dehydration. She refused to eat and we had to put a feeding tube down her nose. Every day I had to hold her down, scrub her stitches and if her tube fell out I had to hold her down and put it back in. I cried buckets over causing my baby pain. With her second surgery at a year of age, we had to splint her arms for weeks to keep her hands out of her mouth, and my thumb-sucking baby had no way of comforting herself. She cried and cried and I felt like a sadist, deliberately depriving her of her favorite thing when she most needed comfort.

Again, was it anything truly tragic? Did my child die, have a permanent disability or suffer major psychiatric trauma? No, but for me, the whole situation was one hurt after another. I spent large amounts of time and money on counseling in order to come to grips with what was, for me, a traumatic experience.

My point in telling both these stories isn't to make you feel sorry for me. I know that many people who read this book will have true trauma involving violation, loss, violence or deliberate neglect which make my experiences seem minor. It's like hearing about a divorce—from the outside it is a commonplace event, but if it's your family being torn apart, it is very traumatic. My point in all this is to drive home the fact that any event which our brain perceives as traumatic will cause pain and hurt and often lead to long-term issues with relationships and depression. So whether the event is viewed by the world as a big deal or a small deal, if it leaves you with lasting hurt that impacts your life, it is an emotional wound for you.

Emotions are very, very complex and your emotional reaction to a situation is never wrong—that's why it's called emotion and not logic. What you do with the emotion, how you react and act, is what will determine your happiness in life. We can hang on to the hurt, carrying it around with us like a badge of honor, or we can choose to let go and heal. It's not as simple as it sounds but again, there are tools that you can use to heal those hurts and move into happiness.

Chapter 7
Healing the Hurts

The emotional component of depression is very complicated. It's not logical and therefore it's far harder to just make a change and "stop it." As we explored before, there are multiple triggers for emotional pain including trauma, loneliness, disappointment, past failures and loss of loved ones. There is clearly not a single approach to emotional pain that is always effective, just as there is not a single approach to the chemical side or the mental side of depression. I will briefly mention a few tools that will help but of course, this list is not comprehensive—if these things don't work for you, don't give up. So often in life it is our journey toward wellness and peace that is fulfilling, not just arriving at the destination. Frequently we become frustrated and impatient if we don't see results right away, and miss the growth that is happening because of the struggle. Keep going. Acknowledge yourself for your hard work. Just starting on the path toward wellness and happiness is an amazing accomplishment. Let's look at some of the tools you can use on your journey.

COUNSELING

Yes, yes, I know, you don't want to talk to someone about how you are feeling, especially someone you don't know. But please, keep an open mind and don't skip this short section. There are as many, many types of counseling and if one style doesn't fit you, try another. I was curious how many different recognized forms of psychotherapy or counseling there are, so I started counting. I counted thirty-two types, including cognitive behavioral therapy, couples counseling, art therapy, existential therapy, solution-focused therapy, and psychoanalysis made famous by Freud, just to name a few. There are also different types of counselors and therapists. A psychiatrist is an MD who prescribes medications and does psychotherapy also. A psychologist is a PhD who cannot prescribe medications but focuses on psychotherapy. I reserve the psychiatrist referral for complicated patients who are not responding to medications and appear to have multiple issues going on. I refer to psychologists when I need help with diagnosis of the actual condition we are dealing with plus therapy. Other types of therapists are commonly referred to as counselors, but are still technically mental health therapists. You may see a host of initials after their names such as LCSW (licensed clinical social worker) or LMHC (licensed mental health counselor). Don't worry about all that. The most important part is getting a good recommendation and getting good results.

If you see a counselor and you don't connect or you don't feel that you are making any progress after the first three visits, find a new therapist. You should not be focused on the traumatic event or the negative emotion for more than the first couple of sessions or the first few minutes of each following session. That isn't helpful and just replays that hurtful rerun in your brain over and over. Instead, you should leave the sessions feeling hopeful, with tools to use in real life. You wouldn't keep going to the same hair salon if they kept giving you a bad haircut, so why stay with the same counselor if you don't start seeing changes in your emotional pattern or relationship pattern? To find a counselor you can call your doctor's office or ask around to neighbors and friends for a recommendation. I know a lot of people are embarrassed about seeing a counselor, however I view counseling like I view exercise—everyone in the world can benefit in one way or another. But if you are uncomfortable asking for recommendations just say, "I am trying to help a friend find a good counselor in the area. Have you heard of anyone good?" It's true because you are your own friend, and if you aren't then you need some counseling to work on that!

Some insurance plans cover counseling, and some counselors bill insurance, but sometimes you just have to make the investment out of pocket if it's what you need to heal. What better thing to invest your money in than your own emotional well being and happiness?

HANDS-ON THERAPIES

In addition to talk therapies, there are also a host of healing therapies involving some form of physical contact or touch that will bring fantastic results. I will quickly run through a few that you can choose from.

- **Biofeedback** helps us become more in tune with and in control of our bodies. Neurofeedback is the same premise for our brain activity. Both of these therapies use monitoring equipment to provide immediate feedback on current conditions in the body or brain, thus allowing us to watch what is effective in changing those conditions. Basically, they are tools that teach us how to be in control of the way our body or brain is functioning.

- **Emotional Freedom Technique** or **"Tapping"** is a unique therapy that involves using your own fingers to tap on certain points and release negative thoughts or limiting beliefs. Yes, that sounds vague and slightly weird, but let me tell you about the power of EFT. After my youngest had her surgeries, I was sad all the time. I was depressed and anxious despite medications, I cried every day, and couldn't let go of the pain, grief and guilt surrounding the situation. I had already seen two counselors without results, but found a counselor who used EFT at my first visit. I broke down and cried, but actually felt lighter for the first time in a year, and I also felt hopeful. The results were immediate and lasting. More and more therapists are integrating this into their practices with fantastic results for patients.

- **Craniosacral therapy** is a treatment that uses slight pressures on the bones of the skull and spine to encourage subtle movements. The theory is that the movements help to restore balance to the nervous system including the signals of the brain. It is frequently used with somato-emotional release, which is the technique of releasing emotional energy stored in the tissue of our bodies. These treatment modalities have far fewer studies backing them up than the others I have listed, but they are extremely soothing and I have seen tremendous healing with patients who utilize this type of therapy.

- **Acupuncture** has been effective for thousands of years for a host of medical issues. Many people know about it as a treatment for pain, but that is just the tip of the iceberg. It is fantastic for depression, anxiety, insomnia, menopause, and allergies among other things. Acupuncture helped me with fertility, pregnancy complications and post-partum complications in addition to my anxiety and depression. I can't say enough good things about acupuncture, and you should treat yourself to a visit if you've never been.

You can Google whichever treatment interests you and find a practitioner near you. Sometimes these things will be covered by insurance but not always, so be sure to clarify before you go.

SELF HELP

I talked about counseling but there is also a lot of emotional healing that we can do within ourselves. One of the most powerful books I've ever read is *Letting Go: The Pathway of Surrender* by David Hawkins, MD. It's a brilliant look at how we can change our emotional state by looking at the energy involved with positive and negative emotions. He guides the reader through the process of letting go of negative emotions and moving into a healing, positive state. That book alone has helped many people I know let go of their pain, trauma and depression.

Personal development seminars are another lovely way of moving out of pain, creating more self esteem and committing to a goal. Depending upon what area of life you want to work on there are a multitude of options you can choose from. The Wings program, PSI, Clearmind, and Tony Robbins Seminars are a few I have seen help people move into action and change. I just attended a Core Strength seminar that is geared toward developing attributes that are key for success, such as confidence or commitment, but a magical thing happened, as often does as development seminars. There were people who came to work on their businesses or sales abilities but instead chose to focus on their emotional healing. I saw several people let go of deep emotional wounds and traumatic memories they had carried for decades.

True healing happens when we are ready to help ourselves. When you are committed to change the way will open up for you to heal.

SPIRITUALITY

We can never truly separate our mind, body and spirit. They are all intertwined, but I find that many people are comfortable talking about mind and body but not so comfortable talking about spirit. Too often people equate spirituality with religion and shy away from exploring this side of themselves. When we neglect our spirituality, we rob ourselves of so much healing power. Have you ever felt that emptiness inside? Some people try to fill it with distractions and pleasure, some try to fill it with drugs or alcohol or power, some try to fill it with food. But none of those things will ever leave you feeling truly whole. Because that emptiness, I believe, is a hole the shape of divinity. If you don't know what you believe about divinity, then I would invite you to explore it. I don't care what religion you practice or if you are completely agnostic—all of us are connected to a greater power, the energy that moves the universe. It could be deity or it could be nature that you connect with, but the point is to make a true connection. Fill that hole inside of you with the divine and it will bring you peace and healing.

We have to develop our spirituality with conscious effort. And I say "develop" because our spirituality is just like our mentality and physicality. You don't get fit and tone by just sitting around. No, you have to develop your muscles through effort and discipline. The same is true of our minds. We don't gain knowledge and intelligence by watching sit-coms and reality TV. No, we have to read, watch educational shows, surround ourselves with mentors. The same is true of our spirituality: it takes work to develop.

I realize that this section will make some uncomfortable, but it's a hugely important part of life and happiness. There are many names used for the divinity in our lives: God, Source Matter, Nature, Energy of the Universe, Goddess. Whatever name you choose, you will start to connect with that energy that unites us all, creates us all and is present in our lives. I personally don't know how I would have survived without my relationship with God. I gain great strength from church attendance and by turning to scripture and prayer for connection with a loving Father in Heaven. But what works for me doesn't work for others, and I encourage you to find what works for you. There are many people who have a relationship with deity without attending church, and many people have spiritual relationships with the higher power of the universe but do not worship a deity at all. You can develop your spirituality in many, many different ways.

One important way you can tap into your spirituality is through meditation. This ancient and powerful practice helps you receive guidance from the universe. It is a way to let go of the past and the future and be present in the now. When I am depressed I am focused too much in the past, weighed down with regret or sadness. When I am anxious I am too worried about tomorrow and what might happen. One of the keys to happiness is to live in the present, the "gift" of the now. Groucho Marx expressed this perfectly when he said, "I have just one day, today, and I'm going to be happy in it." That can be very, very challenging. Meditation is a fabulous tool that can help you not only to open yourself to guidance but also rid yourself of the worries and cares of yesterday and tomorrow and be present in the now. That is a critical skill for living in true happiness. Now, I say all this and admit that I am still a novice at meditation and have found it to be one of the most difficult things to do—likely because you don't "do" anything during meditation. You learn to just "be." And as you learn to be, suddenly you can be connected to that spiritual force that creates and guides and loves all of us.

I have friends who practice yoga daily as their spiritual exercise as well as physical exercise. Many people develop their spirituality by connecting to nature, and still others tap into their divinity by helping others through community service. If you don't know where to start, observe the happiest person you know and find out how they tap into their spiritual strength. Again, there is no one perfect way for everyone to develop their spirituality, but I encourage you to try. You don't expect to go to the gym for the first time and come home looking like a fitness instructor, so please don't expect yourself to reach out for your spiritual connection and have perfect communication right away. Give it time. But I will say that the journey itself toward spirituality is very healing and gives us hope during times of depression and anxiety. I'm so excited for you to get to know all parts of yourself: mental, physical and spiritual. You will find peace in knowing who you truly are, and what is true happiness if not peace with ourselves?

PART 4

THE SPECIAL CIRCUMSTANCES

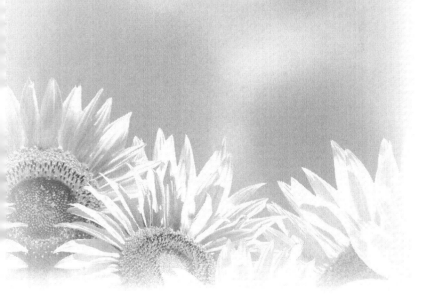

Chapter 8
Anxiety

I have talked about anxiety a lot in this book because often depression and anxiety go hand in hand due to low serotonin. That is not always the case, however. I want to talk a bit about what causes anxiety and how to manage it.

WHY DO YOU FEEL ANXIOUS?

Have you had that uncomfortable feeling of a tight chest, feeling like you can't get enough air? Or the certainty that you are going to die or that something horrible is going to happen? If so you have had the not-so-lovely experience of a panic attack. Most of the time, though, anxiety presents as restlessness, difficulty concentrating, feeling fidgety with the nearly compulsive desire to be moving or doing something. There is often an overall feeling of dread, as though something horrible is about to happen any moment. Why do we feel that way? Of course I'm going to simplify but in short, I explain anxiety this way: Anxiety happens when your brain is over excited and your body responds by producing too much adrenaline. Adrenaline, also known as epinephrine, is your fight-or-flight hormone that is there to keep you safe. In reality, there is not much physical danger in the average life these days, but the psychological stressors we endure daily are perceived by our brain as "dangerous." This triggers adrenaline production as a protective mechanism so we can either run away from the stress or fight the threat. Unfortunately we can do neither, so we sit, day after day, stewing in our stress and adrenaline. Without an outlet for the adrenaline we end up living in a hyper-vigilant state all the time. In other words, we feel anxious. Sometimes there are very logical reasons why we feel anxious and we understand where the anxiety is coming from—a looming deadline, an overdrawn bank account, a very sick child, looking for a job, an overwhelming schedule, etc. Sometimes, though, the cause for our anxiety isn't clear, which then makes us feel more anxious.

So why does our brain get overexcited or why do we produce an excess of adrenaline? There are basically three main reasons. The first reason is a medical condition, and I encounter this the least often. For instance, an adrenaline tumor or a hyperactive thyroid gland would cause anxiety. There are also many medications that can trigger anxiety as a side effect, not to mention the stimulants many people depend on such as coffee and tobacco. I won't go into the illegal stimulants such as cocaine or methamphetamine, but they definitely need to be considered if someone has anxiety that is out of control.

The second reason is a psychiatric condition, meaning you feel anxious because of the changes in your brain chemistry due to depression, bipolar disorder, schizophrenia or some other mental illness. The anxiety in these situations is hard to get under control if the main psychiatric condition such as the bipolar disorder or schizophrenia isn't addressed first. Generalized anxiety disorder is another psychiatric condition and it has its own special considerations.

This third category of primary, or pure anxiety not related to any other condition is a bit more complex than the other two. There is no clear physical or medical condition to cause the anxiety, but there is still anxiety. It's a grinding low level of nervousness and dread that is either there all the time or just pops up in certain situations. The triggers for this anxiety can reside in our subconscious. We can be feeling happy, life is fine on the surface, but we start feeling anxious. If this is the case you need to ask yourself, "What is my subconscious trying to tell me?" It could be that your subconscious is screaming at you to get out of an unhealthy relationship or job, but you keep ignoring it. The brain is our most powerful organ and it will find a way to be heard. If you won't consciously recognize what it's trying to tell you, it will trigger changes in the body that lead to unpleasant symptoms. A rise in adrenaline that leads to a pounding heart and shortness of breath is a classic example. You can read more about this mind–body connection in one of my favorite books, *Heal Your Body A-Z* by Louise Hay.

There are times when just acknowledging the warning from our subconscious is enough to defuse the anxiety. For instance, I used to feel terribly anxious every time I had to ride in the car in the winter. I would sit and chew my fingernails and rub my sweaty palms together. As I got older and asked myself what was going on, I realized that my subconscious was screaming in fear because of the terrible auto accident I was involved in as a small child in slick winter driving conditions. Once I "listened" to my subconscious and pulled the fear out into the open, I was able to reassure myself consciously, which allowed my subconscious to quiet down and stop triggering that anxiety response in the car.

That was a straightforward situation but many people have far more complex subconscious messages related to trauma. I've met people who had chronic anxiety that was only resolved through work that allowed them to visualize an event that happened while they were still in the womb. I've met others who had multiple triggers that seemed completely unrelated to a past trauma, but which their subconscious had somehow lumped together as a threat. I also have a friend who had major anxiety regarding relationships, the source of which stemmed from her great-grandmother's terrible experiences. This is called trans-generational or multi-generational trauma. Clearly it wasn't something she could just talk herself out of logically. It took a lot of work on her part and a lot of help from various sources to get to the root of her subconscious fears.

Again, like our body producing adrenaline to help us fight or run away, our subconscious produces the fear and anxiety to be helpful in warning us about a situation it views as dangerous. Often just by acknowledging what the subconscious is trying to tell us and getting it out in the open starts calming the anxious feelings.

CALMING THE ANXIETY

So how do we address the conscious or subconscious fears so we can lead a life of peace and happiness?

I won't attempt to list everything used in treating anxiety, but I will run through the basics so you have a few tools to choose from.

- **Exercise:** There is absolutely nothing more effective than exercise for both long term anxiety and the occasional panic attack. Exercise allows your body to burn through that adrenaline that causes the "fight or flight" response in your brain, which allows it to calm. You will feel more relaxed, focused and calm after you exercise. It's like a big dose of tranquilizer for your system.

- **Supplements:** Calming that over-excited brain chemistry will be very helpful, and there are a few things that are particularly effective. I have had great results with the homeopathic remedies of Calms or Calms Forte made by Hyland, as well as the supplements L-theanine, inositol, vitamin B6, glutamine, methylated folic acid, and even 5HTP. You can refer to the back index for more details on doses.

- **Meditation:** Even if you are a beginner, even if you have very few moments in the relaxed mindfulness, there will still be huge benefits to meditation. You will notice changes in your perception, your attitude, and your body will change how it responds to stress on a physical level. I promise you will feel better. Just try it. You can Google "meditation for beginners" if you don't know where to start.

- **Self Care:** There are many different ways to approach the physical, mental and spiritual aspects of anxiety. You could see a counselor, a life coach or an angel medium. You can get neurofeedback, massage or acupuncture. You can get your chakras balanced, go on a yoga retreat, or try a nutritional cleanse. Any and all of these have the potential to help, depending upon your personal openness. Start where you are comfortable, but start somewhere.

- **Prioritize:** Life can be incredibly busy with multiple important demands on our time. Instead of trying to complete your whole to-do list every day, just realize that you will only get the first three or four things done. Decide which three or four things are the most important. If you can't decide then ask yourself, "What will matter in a year from now? In five years from now?" Clearly things like your children, relationships and health will pop to the top of the list. After that you can continue to see what is most pressing and urgent, but try and set realistic expectations about what you can accomplish in one day. And if you truly have to get it all done, ask for help!

- **Address your problem head on:** In many cases, anxiety happens because we are avoiding the real issue. Instead of getting our project done or doing the work, we skip out and watch a movie, which creates stress later. Instead of having the hard conversation and setting boundaries, we avoid the short term pain and instead live in long-term dysfunction and stress, creating anxiety. Instead of sitting down and creating a budget, we avoid that stress by doing a little shopping, blowing our budget and creating more anxiety. Often our anxiety is created because we are avoiding the work we need to be doing in order to have a healthy, happy life. Get to work and you will feel better.

- **Pets and Plants:** Nature is a fabulous tranquilizer and two of her best helpers are plants and animals. If you have a pet, bask in the unconditional love and joy of your dog or the entertainment of watching your cat play hard to get. If you don't have a pet, then consider adopting one if circumstances allow. They are breathing bundles of therapy. The other low maintenance option is a plant. Or several plants. House plants can be very rewarding as you watch them grow, literally filling your air with life and if you can get outside and get your hands into the dirt, even better.

Chapter 9
Self Medicating and Addiction

Wouldn't it be great if we all got the help we needed when we needed it? If we all developed healthy coping strategies to use when we were stressed? Unfortunately we don't live in that fairytale land. So what happens when we have depression and anxiety or other mental health issues and we don't get the help we need? Often, we are exposed to chronic stress without learning coping tools—so we develop our own, less-than-healthy coping strategies. We find ways of self-medicating our pain and unhappiness. The self-medication can be as benign an escape mechanism as TV, or as destructive as self-mutilation or illegal drug use.

Too often people without any mental health issues don't understand how anyone could end up destroying their lives with an unhealthy habit. What they don't understand is that no one deliberately destroys their life. Of course no one says, "I would like to become an addict." What happens is we feel terrible—depressed, anxious, confused and filled with self-loathing to the point that we can't function and we are looking for a way to feel better. It starts out very simply as a way to ease the pain for one moment. It feels so good that you end up craving the pleasure as well as the escape from your anxiety and depression.

I've never met an alcoholic or addict who hadn't initially begun using as a way to treat their mental illness, such as anxiety, depression, bipolar disorder, schizophrenia or untreated ADHD. Of course it's not a conscious or logical decision. It is just something that happens as people look for a way to treat the physical issues in their brain chemistry, quiet the mental chatter and fill the spiritual void in their lives. The addiction can be to a drug but it can also be addiction to the release that comes from self-harming.

When I was in residency I was called to the Emergency Department to stitch up a patient. She had multiple deep slices on her arm and I also noticed her other arm had thin white scars covering it. She confessed she cut herself to feel better. "After I cut myself I feel calmer, more peaceful and the voices in my head are quiet." She wasn't talking about hallucinations of voices, she was talking about the negative self-hate thoughts she lived with daily. Cutting gave her a way to punish herself while at the same time exerting control over her life. I've heard bulimics describe their purging in similar terms.

It's heartbreaking to watch a loved one live a life controlled by addiction. My dear little sister led a life controlled by her addiction to pain medication for years. Of course she didn't start out with that end result in mind, but she did want a way to escape from the physical pain of her chronic illness, the emotional pain of a traumatic childhood event, and the mental pain of feeling as though she had failed somewhere along the way. Her narcotic use slowly escalated to the point that she couldn't hide it. I was home on vacation during residency and saw her drop a pill, which bounced across the porch and fell through the slats onto the dirt below. She raced down to dig through the dirt, muttering, "I'm so screwed if I don't find that pill." When I found out it was a narcotic she was digging for I said, "Sis, you have a problem." She initially denied it, became defensive about it and was not grateful at that moment for my opinion. You can't help an addict if they don't want to be helped. That is the hard truth. Fortunately for my sister she had a supportive husband and family and she made the choice to check herself into rehab; she has now been clean for over fifteen years. I'm so proud of her and have learned so much about addiction from watching her journey.

All really good addiction recovery programs include treating not just the physical addiction, but also the mental and spiritual component of addiction. Alcoholics Anonymous is an extremely effective program because it does address all of these areas, connects addicts to a community and gives purpose and value to the lives of those in recovery. If you are struggling with addiction of some kind, please get help. There are free programs, in-patient programs, day programs, doctor supervised programs. Talk to your doctor about your options and remember that there is nothing to be ashamed of and you are not alone in your addiction.

You may not be physically addicted to a substance, but is there an area of your life that you wallow in as an escape? We often look at addicts and alcoholics and feel pity, or relief that we aren't in that position, but if we look more closely at our lives we may realize that we have our own form of addiction: the addiction of avoidance. I certainly struggle with that addiction, for years escaping into books and movies instead of facing my issues and living my life fully.

For example, let's look at the normal activities of shopping, watching TV or movies, eating, sleeping and using social media. All of these things are lovely and often necessary, but if done excessively we miss living our lives in awareness. We become addicted to escaping our lives, which creates a whole set of problems in the health, financial or relationship arenas. Compulsive shopping to escape can lead to debt. Too much time in front of a TV or movies will suck up precious time better spent with loved ones or working on your own life. Turning to food for comfort has caused a health epidemic in our country, and spending our lives napping and oversleeping actually causes more stress because of all the things we don't get done during those hours

As I said, none of those is in itself a bad thing, but they can become unhealthy if used as an escape. The question to ask yourself is, "Am I happy in my life? Am I living it fully or am I finding ways to escape?" If you are escaping for hours every week, odds are you aren't truly happy.

Chapter 10
Young children and teens

Children and teens are not just little adults. They have their own sets of challenges and their brains are not fully developed. There is nothing more troubling as a parent than to watch one of my children feel unhappy. When it happens chronically and a child is depressed or very anxious it is very painful for both parent and child. This is the time to connect with your child and also ask for help from your physician. Let's look at each group individually.

YOUNG CHILDREN

It's rare for young children to be inherently depressed if they have had a happy childhood and a healthy family. But again, what are healthy and happy? As we discussed before, everyone has baggage from childhood and there is no truly "normal" family since we all have our quirks and traditions. For the most part, though, it's uncommon to find a clinically depressed child in an otherwise happy family with no history of mental illness or depression, unless the child has experienced trauma. Children overall have the gift of joy.

That being said, we are all influenced by our surroundings and genetics and children can, and do, become depressed. Depression in children often looks different than in adults. A child with depression can appear hyperactive, antisocial, and argumentative rather than down and sad. In addition, children can become anxious. Yes, anxiety and depression are two sides of the same coin of low serotonin, but anxiety can also be a product of a stressful environment. If a child grows up with an anxious parent who frets and worries constantly and can never fully relax, then the child can start behaving the same way, subconsciously believing there is a reason to behave in a fearful manner. The reverse is also true—if children witness their parents dealing with stress in a calm fashion then they will learn some of those healthy coping behaviors.

If you have a child who is appearing anxious, depressed or chronically unhappy in some fashion I would always suggest starting with plenty of reassurance and one-on-one time with your child, but I would also recommend an appointment with your pediatrician or family doctor just to be sure there isn't anything else going on. There are a variety of medical conditions that can lead to anxiety, including food allergies, sensory integration disorder, sleep apnea and some genetic disorders. A physician will also screen for abuse so don't be offended or fearful if that is brought up during the visit.

On the whole, children are very resilient and tend to respond extremely well to extra love and attention in times of stress. In addition to that, there are a few tools that are fantastic for any parent to use with their children. I personally love the Integrated Listening System or ILS. It helps with self-calming and self regulation and it is fantastic for both kids and adults, especially in the setting of anxiety. There is also a variety of over-the-counter homeopathic remedies, including Hyland brand Calms and Calms forte. I also love the magnesium powder that can be used to make a fizzy drink at bedtime—it helps with restlessness and some patients report it helps leg cramps. Essential oils are another fantastic tool. A couple of drops of lavender on the pillow case or behind the ears is a lovely place to start. Again, please don't try a bunch of different remedies in lieu of a medical evaluation, but you can safely try these on children five years of age or older. Lavender oil on the pillow case is fine for a child of any age.

The most important thing to remember is that you know your child better than anyone, so never ignore your gut instincts. If you follow your parenting intuition and let love lead you, you can never do the wrong thing for your child.

TEENS

I have a passion for adolescent medicine and in my practice I see a lot of teens with depression, anxiety or sleep issues. Sometimes these issues pop up because they inherited the brain chemistry that sets them up for depression or they have an untreated condition such as attention deficit disorder or a low thyroid. Apart from the physical component, though, there is always the mental and emotional component of their lives that can lead to depression. Teens may have experienced a trauma such as abuse, neglect, or homelessness, but that is less often than the chronic social and emotional stressors of being a teen. The bottom line is that, like with adults, depression in teens is a combination of the physical, mental and spiritual stressors in their lives, and all these areas need to be addressed in order to optimally transition them into a happier place in life.

Too often their parents are more interested in getting these teens help than they are themselves. Sound familiar? Don't despair. I would say the first step is to call around and find a doctor who enjoys treating depressed or anxious teens. The appropriate question would be "Does Doctor X see a lot of teens with depression or anxiety in his practice and does he have a few different counselors that he refers to?" You want someone who has a network of different providers to refer his or her teen patients out to for counseling, which is a hugely important part of treatment. You can have them see a psychiatrist or you can start with your family doctor or pediatrician, which is less intimidating for most teens, as well as a more relaxed environment.

So what if you have a kid who just refuses to be seen or won't cooperate? There are a couple of things that have worked for me and my patients. The first is to make an appointment for a check-up, or for a specific issue such as fatigue or sleep issues or appetite issues, and let the doctor know ahead of time your concerns. You can do this either through a letter, email or phone call, or even talking with him or her outside the room prior to the appointment. It really helps me as a doctor to have a heads up about what is going on, and it lets me know to work around to depression screening. I never jump right in and ask, "Are you depressed?" That makes them close up for sure. I ask about sleep, appetite, energy, and mood, and then explain that depression is due to chemical changes in our brain that we can work on together. I enroll them into the treatment process by asking them if they would like to feel better and what they would be willing to do in order to feel better. You can never force a teenager to do anything long term.

There are some teens who know they are depressed and refuse to go to the doctor or counselor, or refuse to speak during an appointment. It's up to the provider to get them to come out of their shell, but as a parent I would suggest finding your child's "currency." Meaning, what will motivate your teen? I promise, there is something. Money, car privileges, new computer game, and don't forget, one-on-one time with you is a surprisingly strong motivator. You can ask them directly if you don't know. They will shrug and act like nothing matters, but keep observing and you will figure it out. That is the carrot approach to the situation and sometimes it needs to be combined with the stick, meaning loss of privileges. Most teens have a cell phone or iPod or something of the sort. Those are privileges that can be revoked if they aren't cooperative. I'm not saying be a dictator, I'm just saying be up front about your desire to help them feel better and you will do your part and if they do theirs they will earn whatever their currency is. If they don't, they will lose a privilege for a few days. One last thing: I cannot emphasize enough that you do not want them isolating themselves in their room with a TV or a computer. A TV in the bedroom is never going to lead to anything good, but rather causes sleep issues and isolates people from their families. The goal is to get your teen out of their room and interacting as much as possible.

I would also find way to help them interact with the community as well. It can be taking part in extracurricular activities or church activities but also think about community service. Taking your teenager with you to serve food at the homeless shelter or help in a nursing home is a great way of getting them out of their own heads and helping them appreciate what they do have. As we talked about, gratitude is a fantastic antidote to unhappiness.

Again, teens are complex, with a mixture of physical, hormonal and social pressures. In addition to those normal issues there can be the added complication of recreational drugs. It is something that always has to be considered with abrupt behavior or mood changes, and if your doctor doesn't talk to you about it, please bring it up yourself if you have concerns. If the first doctor or counselor doesn't work, find a new one. A good doctor is a bit like a good hairstylist—you are going to ask around, observe who looks good and try them out. If it's not a good fit, start over.

Most important of all with teens, they have this complex push–pull behavior. They pretend not to want your rules, guidance or presence in their lives and push you away, but subconsciously they crave the security that comes from knowing someone loves them enough to give them structure. Subconsciously they are pulling you toward them, craving unconditional love. Let them know they have that with you and most of all, don't give up on them.

Chapter 11

Pregnancy and Postpartum Depression

Pregnancy and the first few months of your newborn's life are exciting and wonderful times, and a cause for great celebration and joy. They are also the cause of great amounts of heartache and discomfort for some. The focus of these times is understandably on your infant, but it is very important to take care of yourself as well, not just physically but also mentally and emotionally. Let's cover the two time periods separately, since they have different issues associated with them.

PREGNANCY

The Depression Health Center of WebMD states that one in four women will experience depression at one point or another in their lives. We are particularly susceptible to depression during pregnancy. There are a few causes for this, including the wild changes in hormone levels and the fatigue from growing another human being inside your body. In addition, many women have increased stress in their lives during pregnancy, such as relationship or financial stressors. Previous miscarriages, complications with the current pregnancy and infertility make depression much more likely. If you are already predisposed to depression, it is more likely to make an appearance during pregnancy.

If you look at a list of symptoms of depression in pregnancy, it may make you laugh, since half of the symptoms are normal for an expectant mother. What woman doesn't have changes in her sleep patterns and eating patterns, as well as changes in libido? That being said, if your sleep and appetite issues are extreme and making it hard to function, it's time to mention them to your doctor. More importantly, if you are having issues with feeling sad or hopeless, or are struggling with thoughts of death or suicide, you need to be seen immediately.

If you are starting to feel depressed, there are a couple of things that will help you during this time. The first is regular gentle exercise and the second is good nutrition and adequate rest. I would also suggest seeing a counselor or at least plugging into your support system regularly. Counseling is as effective as medication for mild to moderate depression. Speaking of which, medications definitely pose risks to your unborn child, but if you need a prescription drug, there are a couple that are safer than others and your doctor can talk to you about your options. Severe untreated depression during pregnancy can lead to complications with your baby's growth as well as the delivery and post-partum period.

I don't usually recommend supplements for expectant moms just because we don't have enough information on the safety of most of them during pregnancy. I would talk to your doctor about any supplements you are considering. There are a few essential oils that are safe, such as lavender and the citrus oils, but other than that make sure you talk with your doctor about any other treatments. This is a magical time and if you aren't able to enjoy it then it's time for a change. You are about to meet the new little life you have cradled within you for months!

POSTPARTUM DEPRESSION

There are so many resources focused on preparing women for the process of childbirth, but relatively few focused on the post-partum period. I find that interesting, since recovering from a delivery while dealing with plummeting hormones, sleepless nights and shifting relationships is amazingly demanding. Yes, delivery is a grueling process but it only lasts a few hours, or if you are unlucky, a couple of days. The first part of your baby's life lasts months and has its own set of unique challenges.

I remember when I was pregnant with my oldest, and my best friend from med school called me. She had her first baby in our last year of medical school. She said, "Remember how tired you were during internship when you were working 100 hours a week? That is a piece of cake compared to the sleep deprivation you are about to experience." I laughed, not understanding that she was dead serious. No one can fully explain the sleep deprivation that is experienced with a new baby.

I was so excited to meet my daughter, especially since we had struggled with fertility. I had waited so long for a baby and, like many women who struggle with fertility, I had been idealizing life with a newborn. In my head I was picturing a wonderful natural birth followed by a peaceful time full of snuggling and bonding, tranquil breast feeding and a cooing happy baby. In short, I had grossly unrealistic expectations. My sweet daughter came into life via a cesarean section, which dashed my dreams of a natural delivery and caused its own grief. She also came with strong opinions and colic, which didn't help my crashing hormones and ridiculous fatigue. I distinctly remember reaching the breaking point. One night my husband was at work at the fire station and I had just gotten my fussy baby to sleep. I was dying for a treat to pick me up and dished up a bowl of chocolate ice cream. Just as I lifted the spoon to my mouth she let out a loud screech and started wailing. An hour later I finally got her back to sleep and I came back to the kitchen to find my bowl of ice cream melted to a puddle of brown goop. I started to cry. "I can't even plan to eat a bowl of ice cream. My life is totally out of my control!" Looking back, after three kids, I laugh because of course life is out of control with a newborn. They are tiny tyrants who control you completely. But for me it was a huge change that I wasn't ready for, and it sent my anxiety into the stratosphere. That soon spiraled into depression.

True post-partum depression affects between 12-20 percent of women, whereas the "baby blues" are much more common. The difference is the severity and duration of symptoms. If you are experiencing symptoms of depression that interfere with your ability to function and/or the symptoms last longer than two weeks, it's more than just crashing hormones and sleep deprivation. It's full-on depression and you need to be seen. Your doctor or midwife should be screening you for depression—the Edinburgh postpartum screening tool is the most commonly used questionnaire and does a good job of picking up on depression in new moms.

If you are breast feeding your baby then you are limited in what you can take for your mood as far as supplements and medication, for the same reasons as during pregnancy. I would again start with counseling, exercise, nutrition, light therapy and getting as much sleep as possible. Please ask for help and let people watch your baby so you can nap. If things are getting worse instead of better, definitely talk to your doctor, because there are a few medications for depression that are safe to take while breastfeeding.

Awareness of postpartum depression has greatly improved, thanks in part to a couple brave celebrity moms airing the issue to the public. In the past there was definitely shame attached to postpartum depression and a woman was made to feel unnatural if she was sad, overwhelmed or if she had thoughts of harming herself or her baby. Fortunately there is more understanding about this significant issue and there are more resources available. Mom support groups are one of the best tools available to you if you have postpartum depression. Remember, you are not alone in this issue, there are people waiting to help you.

Chapter 12
Wrapping it up

As I said in the beginning, this book is not meant to be a comprehensive resource for treating depression or anxiety, and it certainly doesn't replace medical care. Every person is different, with a different set of genetics, life experiences and brain chemistry. There is never going to be a one-size-fits-all guide to treating illness and sadness, so don't feel hopeless if you are trying the things I've suggested and not seeing results. It doesn't mean you should give up—it just means your journey will take longer than you expected. But is there any journey more worthwhile than the journey of self-discovery and healing? Is there any goal more profound or more exciting to anticipate than wellness? As you are on your journey, I want you to remember that your mind, body and spirit are intertwined and you cannot heal one without addressing the other two.

No matter what your circumstances are, you can change them. It may be that you got dealt a terrible hand by life and grew up in an abusive family, or have a strong genetic predisposition toward depression or have experienced major trauma at some point; none of these things have the power to control your life unless you let them. Up to this point you have created your reality by accepting the story you tell yourself about your life. These stories we tell ourselves are called limiting beliefs. They are beliefs, not realities, about our lives that limit us. For example, I told myself for years that I would always struggle with depression because of the strong family genetics I had inherited. That limited my efforts in looking for ways to feel better.

I also had the horrible realization that I wanted to be depressed more than I wanted to be happy. You might ask, why I would have such a sick desire? Because as a depressed person I was excused from trying something new, from pushing myself and from taking risks. Basically, my depression was my safe zone. Ask yourself, do you have a subconscious reward for holding on to your depression? Is it attention? Is it a buffer from possible failure?

There are many things that can hold us back from wellness, whether it's the beliefs we embrace as truth or the subconscious rewards we find in our role as a "sick person". The bottom line is that we have to make the decision to change our circumstances. Jen Sincero, in her brilliant book *You are a Badass*, puts it best when she says, "If you're serious about changing your life, you'll find a way. If you're not, you'll find an excuse." Are you finding a way or are you finding an excuse? I have absolute faith in you that you will find a way. I'm privileged to be part of your journey and can't wait to hear about your shift from depression to happiness. May you find peace in the journey and embrace each moment as it comes.

Supplements

This is a very short index of the supplements I mentioned in the book. It is by no means a comprehensive list of all the supplements available to help with mood disorders.

FOR DEPRESSION

Multivitamin –high quality

5HTP - Start with 50-100 mg at night; can take up to 100 mg twice a day

Vitamin D3 - 1,000-5,000 units a day

St. John's Wort - Start 300 mg daily, work up to 300 mg three times a day if needed

FOR ANXIETY

L-Theanine – 100 mg twice a day

Glutamine - 500-1,500 mg three times a day

GABA - 100–500 mg three times a day

B6 – 50 mg daily

FOR DEPRESSION OR ANXIETY

L-methylfolate - 7–15 mg daily

Inositol - Start 2,000 mg twice a day, work up to 6,000 mg three times a day

FOR SLEEP

5HTP -100 mg at bedtime

Melatonin – 1 mg to start, and increase to maximum of 5 mg

Calms Forte by Hyland - 1–3 tablets a day

Additional Resources

National Institute of Mental Health website:
www.nimh.nih.gov

Anxiety and Depression Association of America website:
www.adaa.org

UCLA Free Guided Meditations website:
http://marc.ucla.edu/body.cfm?id=22

The Depression Cure by Stephen S. Ilardi

Prescription for Natural Cures by James F. Balch M.D., Mark Stengler N.M.D., Robin Young Balch N.D.

Exercise for Mood and Anxiety, by Michael W. Otto and Jasper A. J. Smits

Bibliography

Andrews, Andy. *Traveler's Gift: Seven Decisions that Determine Personal Success.* Nashville, W. Publishing Group, 2002

Elrod, Hal. *Miracle Morning: The Not-So-Obvious Secret Guaranteed to Transform Your Life Before 8 AM.* United States, Hal Elrod International, 2012

Emoto, Masaru. *Hidden Messages in Water.* Hillsboro, Beyond Words Publishing, 2004

Hawkins, David. *Letting Go: The Pathway of Surrender.* United States, Hay House, 2013

Hay, Louise L. *Heal Your Body A-Z,* New York, Hay House, Inc. 1998

Helmstetter, Shad. *What to Say When You Talk to Yourself.* New York, Pocket Books, 1982

Hill, Napoleon. *Think and Grow Rich.* United States, Wilder Publication, Reprint 2007.

Losier, Michael. *Law of Attraction: The Science of Getting More of What You Want, Less of What You Don't.* New York, Hachette Book Group, 2003

Pollan, Michael. *In Defense of Food: An Eater's Manifesto.* New York, Penguin Press, 2008

Scott, Trudy. *Antianxiety Food Solution.* Oakland: New Harbinger Publications, 2011

Sincero, Jen. *You Are a Badass: How to Stop Doubting Your Greatness and Start Living an Awesome Life.* Philadelphia, Running Press, 2013

Seuss. *Oh, The Places You'll Go!,* United States, Random House, 1960

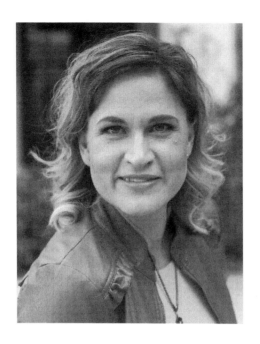

Dr. Raphael Allred has a busy private practice as a family physician and she emphasizes holistic treatment options with her patients. Over the last 15 years of practice she has developed a passion for empowering her patients through education and allowing them to make informed decisions about their health care. Her practice focus is on mental health, nutrition and preventive medicine. She lives with her family in Bend, Oregon.

Notes

Notes

Notes

Notes

Notes

Notes

42981206R00062

Made in the USA
San Bernardino, CA
12 December 2016